turning **FAT** into **LOVE**

# turning FAT into LOVE

### Downsize Your Body by
### Supersizing Your Mind & Heart

## PAULINE KERKHOFF

NEW YORK

# turning FAT into LOVE
## Downsize Your Body by Supersizing Your Mind & Heart

Published in New York, New York, by Morgan James Publishing. Morgan James and The Entrepreneurial Publisher are trademarks of Morgan James, LLC. www.MorganJamesPublishing.com

The Morgan James Speakers Group can bring authors to your live event. For more information or to book an event visit The Morgan James Speakers Group at www.TheMorganJamesSpeakersGroup.com.

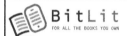

**BitLit**

FOR ALL THE BOOKS YOU OWN

FREE eBook edition for your existing eReader with purchase

PRINT NAME ABOVE

For more information, instructions, restrictions, and to register your copy, go to **www.bitlit.ca/readers/register** or use your QR Reader to scan the barcode:

ISBN 978-1-61448-772-2  paperback
ISBN 978-1-61448-773-9  eBook
ISBN 978-1-61448-774-6  audio
ISBN 978-1-61448-874-3  hardcover
Library of Congress Control Number:
2013946001

**Cover Design by:**
Rachel Lopez
www.r2cdesign.com

**Interior Design by:**
Bonnie Bushman
bonnie@caboodlegraphics.com

In an effort to support local communities, raise awareness and funds, Morgan James Publishing donates a percentage of all book sales for the life of each book to Habitat for Humanity Peninsula and Greater Williamsburg.

Get involved today, visit
www.MorganJamesBuilds.com.

**Habitat for Humanity®**
Peninsula and
Greater Williamsburg
Building Partner

*For Kiki and Daan:*
*My love for you will always support*
*and carry you, no matter what.*
*You will become who you want to be.*
*You will be free to do what you love to do.*
*Just be yourself.*
*Becoming the mother of you two*
*is the greatest gift of my life.*
*Ik hou van jullie, lieve schatjes.*
*Mama*

# CONTENTS

# Introduction

# ANYTHING
# IS POSSIBLE

My father and I stood together in the Ooijpolder Nijmegen in the Netherlands, looking out on the lovely little lake nestled in the beautiful, wide landscape. It was my father's birthday, but we did not feel like celebrating. "You have a future!" my father said exasperatedly, as I stood there sobbing. I had just been diagnosed with relapsing remitting multiple sclerosis (MS).

I was so relieved to be finally getting treatment and to have a name for the cluster of vague symptoms, including the loss of sight, loss of sensitivity, and fatigue that had gotten worse over many years. But at the same time I felt absolutely devastated about my future and the uncertainty of the disease. "You have a future!" my father repeated.

I nodded my head, tears rolling down my face. "I know, Daddy, but not the future as I dreamt of it. I wanted to marry and have kids, and now I will be alone for the rest of my life and I will never become a mother." With that last sentence my heart broke into a thousand pieces, and the silent crying transformed into the real deal, complete with sobs, gasping for air, and a tsunami of water from my eyes and nose.

"Sweetheart," my father said, as he gently stroked my back. "It might not be exactly the future you thought you would have or I thought you would have. But you still have a future. Everybody has a future! You might not be able to have children, but you might consider adopting them. And with your personality and looks you will find love as well. Trust me honey, it will work out fine."

Personality? Looks? Did he forget what the doctor just told us? Did he really think that anyone could care more about my personality than my burden? That anyone could be more interested in what I had to offer than in what I was about to lose? That anyone could be attracted by me, while I felt disgusted by my own body? That anyone would find freedom with me, while I felt held hostage?

My father saved my life by not giving up on me on that day, by seeing a bright happy future for me. A little spark of hope ignited in my heart, and I tried to live from that little spark, even though I could not yet see or believe everything that he saw.

> ♥ Have you ever lost hope for a better future?
> ♥ Do you believe change in your life is necessary, but you feel stuck?
> ♥ Do you want to create your better future now?

Anything is possible, even when everything seems impossible.

Because my father was right: Within three years after this diagnosis, my dreams turned into reality. Not only did I meet a very humorous and attractive man who proposed to me; not only did I start my own business as a nutritionist and dietician to help many people lose weight; but I was also blessed to become the mother of the two most precious gifts of my life, Kiki and Daan.

I was so afraid my MS was going to make me an obstacle to others, but with the birth of my children, two little twinkling stars were planted next to that spark of hope my father had planted in my heart years earlier. By staying very connected to my heart, I am not an obstacle, but I can instead be a beacon for my kids and for others.

Nevertheless, I still occasionally lose hope for my future. During those times I ask myself, *How on earth did I get here, and how do I move on?* One such moment, eleven years after my MS diagnosis, happened during my difficult decision to divorce. I never believed in happily ever after, but I believed in the power of love, and I still do. I also believe, however, that everybody should be able to grow in a relationship, and that kids have the right to a stable and warm home, even if this means being raised by a single parent. It took a lot of courage and faith in a better future for me to make this choice, but even so, anything is possible.

Health and love are so important for your happiness, and sometimes we must lose both to see that importance clearly.

Although the MS has been stable for several years now, I recently went through a period of poor health. As I was going through the divorce, I became overweight—even though I was a nutritionist and dietician and knew exactly how I "should" be eating. The truth was that I was eating to compensate for the lack of love in my life. In other words, I was turning love into fat: I was eating sweet things to feel better, to feel important, to feel rewarded, and even to feel connected to myself. But in the end it turned out to be a coping mechanism that didn't solve the real problem. In fact, it made things worse.

Now, I have discovered that self-love heals pain better than food. I have discovered that consistent self-care coming from within melts more fat than any diet ever can. I have discovered that eating your feelings away, ignoring your health, and hiding from your problems is not the best solution for transforming yourself into the healthy, happy, and loving person you are meant to be.

I have discovered that thinking the wrong way can do a lot of harm. I have discovered that the wrong thoughts can cause wrong feelings, which in turn cause wrong words and actions. In particular, I have discovered that judging your body does not make it slimmer.

I have learned from those mistakes. I have transformed myself, and so can you, if you want. You can turn fat back into love.

In my opinion, love and leadership are the best tools for transforming yourself.

Here's what I mean. Growing love in your heart and taking leadership over your mind and actions will jumpstart your transformation. First you have to accept and love yourself as you are now, and then think, talk, and act in a way that is congruent with your goals and dreams. This book will show you how to feel more love by supersizing your heart, and to show more leadership by growing your brain and upgrading your thinking. The more control you have over your thoughts, actions, and emotions, the more easily your body can be changed.

*Turning Fat into Love* is not a diet. It is not an instant fix for melting your belly fat. It is an exciting long-term project, an adventure that will test your skills and make you experience things previously unknown to you.

Allow me to take you on this journey. Travel with me toward your happier and healthier self. You will explore new tactics, get rid of the old tactics that haven't worked for you, and commit to the new ones that do.

You will investigate your own barriers on your journey and learn how to turn those roadblocks into redirections. You will enjoy personal growth and weight loss at the same time. In other words, you will lose weight not only physically, but also emotionally and mentally.

It is time to switch into high gear on the highway of life and to get rid of all the weight that has been holding you back for too long. It is time to unleash your greatest source of energy and become unstoppable in life. It is time to finally let go of all your fears and your excuses and to let more love in. You deserve that. It is your time, my friend, and I am here to help you. You don't have to be fixed; you are not broken. You are worthy of love no matter your size, income, accomplishments, or looks.

Maybe you already feel happy and healthy, but you want to explore how you can improve yourself. Let me help you become your best, happiest, and healthiest self. And maybe you just are curious about the title of this book: *Turning Fat into Love*—what is that about? I welcome you too, and I honor your curiosity and your openness to new approaches. Promise me one thing: If you are committed to turning fat into love, even more than you believe in this book and this process, believe in yourself, because right now, just as you are, you have everything it takes to become more happy and fit than you have ever been in your life.

I'm going to share my struggles freely with you, so you can hopefully avoid them in your own life. And if you've already gone through them, then we can commiserate together and help each other continue to move forward.

After all, this book has emerged from my own transformative journey, both personally and professionally. I have dealt with illness, divorce, and utter financial destitution. However, I have also discovered that those were not mistakes or failures, but opportunities to grow. And I am so happy with my life. I am not happy in spite of those events; I am happy *because* I had the opportunity to deal with them and overcome them. Learn from my stories, be inspired, and become a beacon for your loved ones. Because you are already, even though you might sometimes feel like you are in the shadows. I will not give up on you, no matter where you are at this moment in your life, dear reader. You should not either.

Supersize your heart, grow your brain, do the high five to improve your life, transform your body, and change the world.

Anything is possible. Even when at times it seems impossible.

# Chapter 1

# SUPERSIZE YOUR HEART

Three or four times a year, I am a mother who loves to bake cookies. The messier the kitchen, the better and tastier the dough. My two-year-old son, Daan, does not like the taste of the dough, but he enjoys cleaning his spot on the kitchen counter. With water. A lot of water. Not my daughter Kiki and I. We love tasting the dough before we begin cutting out the cookies. Afterward everything is spic and span: Daan has cleaned the kitchen counter, and Kiki has licked all the kitchen utensils and pastry bowls clean. That saves me some time and energy in these busy days! (You know I am kidding, right?)

We are proud when the cookies are baked, and we enjoy the taste, smell, and sight of the cookie stars, the puppets, and the little footballs made by Daan. But the most tempting are the hearts, decorated with pink glazing and silver sugar pearls. Sometimes we make little holes in the hearts, so we can hang them in the Christmas tree with pretty red ribbons. The hearts with holes in them almost never make it to the Christmas tree; they are usually devoured by little hungry mouths long before they get anywhere near the tree.

Like the heart-shaped cookies, you might feel like you have a hole in your heart, too. You may feel empty, unfulfilled, or restless, without knowing exactly why. Or maybe you do know why. Does it feel as if someone has devoured your heart? Or as if your heart is not whole anymore?

You are not the only one. You are not alone.

Sometime during your life, someone who was not capable of giving you what you needed at that moment may have cut a hole out of your heart, just as if your heart were made of cookie dough. Those holes might be of various shapes and sizes, leaving an emptiness that is not easily filled. Those holes might have the shape of an absent father, a depressed mother, or a boyfriend or girlfriend. Someone who hurt you emotionally years ago may have left a footprint in the dough that is still visible. Your ex may have cut out the shape of a little heart and ate it with gusto. Or someone tried to knead your heart dough in such a way that it never can return to its authentic form.

Life is not always easy when you have a heart with holes in it. Some people try to fill up the holes with working too much, with the Internet, or with alcohol or drugs. But many people try to fill up these holes with food—by eating chocolate, or cookies, or chips, or candy. As if you want to compensate for the feelings of deprivation or the lack of sweetness in your life.

You may find yourself trying to get your heart back into its original shape by eating a lot, quickly, now. Now, because the need to feel better is so urgent you cannot postpone eating. Quickly, because you don't want to get caught in the act. And a lot, because your body will never, ever be able to send you a stop signal. You won't feel a stop signal because your body did not ask for food in the first place and because your hunger is at another level—you are trying to fix an emotional hunger with physical food. You want to fill the holes in your heart by eating, but the food will never get there. Still you keep repeating the same trick: A lot. Quickly. Now. Secretly.

If you want to lose weight long term, you have to make sure that your heart returns to its original big ball of dough. Only then will you not have to turn to food to fill your empty feelings.

Here is my recipe for a big tasty portion of heart dough.

## 1. First Love Yourself before You Fly

If I could teach you one thing, it would be how to transform your heart in such a way that you could feel an abundance of self-love 24/7, because that is the only healthy thing you can do for yourself and your loved ones that will result in lasting change in your life. Consistent self-care starts with self-love. If you think you are not worthy enough, how are you going to take care of yourself in an excellent way? And how can you really empathize with others when you can't tolerate the same fear of failure or feelings of shame within yourself?

In the time leading up to my divorce, my husband was not very affectionate. I found it difficult to love myself. I was tired and felt like a failure. I struggled with my career and I gained weight. My husband's criticism about my business or about the household felt like he had stabbed me in my soul, because I took it personally. To the world I showed confidence, but inside I cried about the lack of control over my own life, and I felt like I was drifting further and further away from my dreams. The lack of sweetness in my daily life had to be compensated for, and I started to eat. In the evening. While reading a book or watching TV or driving in my car. Everything I taught my clients, everything I knew was important about healthy eating, every rule and every piece of advice I had ever given, all best practices diminished into hollow and empty words. I was not walking the talk anymore. Even worse, as a director of a successful weight management institute, I started gaining weight. Very successfully. Because I also received Prednisolon treatments from time to time, I sometimes used that as my excuse for my big belly and fat cheeks. But deep down inside I knew better. I was very good at transforming people into healthier and thus happier people, but I could not help myself.

Sweet candy, meant for children, disappeared in my mouth, but never reached or filled the big hole in my heart— as if my heart were on a diet and did not accept sweetness. Thus began a vicious cycle, which got to the point where I went to the store to buy drop (a Dutch candy) because I felt I could not survive one minute further without instantly filling up my emptiness inside. I had no idea how to connect to self-love, and I felt better after eating the candy. For a little while.

> Do you have moments when you are not thinking about eating at all? Describe them. What are you doing and with whom?

I never ate that much when I was really present with the kids or with friends. I ate their love instead of candy, and it fulfilled me more than anything else. I borrowed their faith in me when I lacked it, and when I looked at myself through their admiring eyes, instead of judging myself, I felt beautiful. I felt beautiful and radiant instead of fat and ugly when I used their eyes as a loving mirror.

If you really want to gain self-respect and self-love instead of gaining pounds, eat some love instead of food. Eat it by borrowing the faith of others and by looking at yourself through their loving, compassionate eyes, and you will feel better. Your self-love will grow instead of your belly. Speak to yourself with a loving voice instead of judging yourself harshly, look to yourself with compassionate eyes, and give to yourself what you try to seek outside yourself. Sometimes people cannot give you what you need at this moment, so learning to give it to yourself helps you progress in life.

---

The moment you feel bad about yourself, try this exercise:

♥ Do you have people around you who love you?

♥ Can you try to look at yourself through their compassionate eyes, instead of your own judging eyes?

♥ What do you see when you look at yourself through their eyes?

♥ If you cannot answer that question, ask them—they will explain why you are so lovable.

---

If you love yourself enough, it is easier to take good care of yourself. Think about how you treat your best friend. Do you take care of yourself the same way? Do you feel you deserve that as well?

You can nurture and nourish yourself so much better than any food ever will.

This next exercise might be not for everybody, but I place it here for those who might benefit.

Imagine that you have a younger self inside you who still craves attention and love and care because she (or he) lacked that. Her needs were not being met, so she remains in a state of feeling small, wanting, deprived, and not having and not being enough.

You have grown up now, but that younger self deep inside you can still dominate your life. Maybe it is time to give her what she needs. She needs your acceptance, your approval, your care, and your seeing that she exists. She does not need chips, chocolate, or cheese—they don't care about her. You should care about her like a parent or caretaker. Feel and be with the pain she experiences; it will not go away when you deny it is there. Calm her, love her, and let her move on. This will take time and effort and perhaps even some therapy. If you need therapy, allow yourself that gift instead of feeling ashamed. You will feel so much better after you have healed those old wounds, after you have healed yourself, so that you finally can become who you truly are. You can become you. You will become more authentic.

## 2. Add 24 Hours of Authenticity per Day

Authenticity is the key to connecting to yourself and others at the highest levels. Being authentic means that you are connected to your own heart and values and that you act congruently with them. You are trustworthy toward yourself and you are genuine. Authentic people don't have to perform to please other people; they choose to be themselves all the time. They are often so in balance that they don't feel particularly better after compliments and no worse after criticism or failure. They share their fears and failures just as easily as their successes.

You might recognize people who are not acting authentic and not being present. You might ask yourself after meeting them, "Why do I feel so hollow or even cheated when this person is only being nice to me?" It is the salesman asking you how he can help you but is not really interested in your answer, only your money. It is the neighbor who asks how you are doing but is not really looking in your eyes to see the answer. It is the husband who seems to listen when you are so excited about something that you want to share but is really more interested in his iPad.

Not being authentic wastes a lot of energy. Acting like someone else on the stage of life takes a tremendous effort. When you finally choose to be 100 percent authentic, you will be astonished at how much energy you will have. That is because it all happens effortlessly when you are plugged in to the enormous power of your heart and your soul.

Smiley Blanton said, "The truth is that all of us attain the greatest success and happiness possible in this life whenever we use our native capacities to their greatest extent."[1]

What would happen if you allowed all your authentic strengths to become the focus in your life, the center and the foundation of your behavior—so that everything you do is shaped by your unique gifts instead of driven by your problems, and all you do is touched by your love instead of contaminated by your doubts and negative energy?

The answer to all of this lies in you. You need to plug in with your authentic self. Be prepared: when you connect with your authentic self, all of your self will emerge, not only your pretty, happy, and amazing self, but also your darker sides, the parts you have been choosing not to show to the world because you were not proud of them, the parts that you have tried to cover up.

Welcome all of you, your brightest and your darkest sides. Trying to resist your shadows will end up in suffering and thus overeating. You have to learn to accept and honor all these parts of yourself to feel whole again. Embrace your anger, welcome your fears, feel those negative feelings instead of numbing them with food or TV or the Internet or work or alcohol or drugs or whatever. If you are capable of accepting all of you, including your shadows, you will be in balance like you never were before. Some parts of you will be admired and loved by people, and other parts will cause trouble all the time and complicate your life. Learn to accept who you are.

---

1    Source: http://www.quotationspage.com/quote/1948.html.

> ♥ What five words do you want to describe you when you are living up to your highest authentic potential?
>
> ♥ What words describe you now, when you look at your behavior and results in life?

You really are who you repeatedly say you are, so if you keep saying you are shy and weak, others will perceive you as shy. But if you repeatedly say and feel that you are strong, other people (and your own subconscious) will accept that, too! The choice is yours. Be careful with the words you use to describe yourself.

Decide who you want to be from now on and behave congruently with that vision. Don't let your past define you anymore. You are who you want to be, not who you decided to be years ago. You can decide who you want to become at any moment in life. Who do you want to be? Who do you not want to be?

Be proud of who you really are deep inside, and never be afraid to show that person to the world—rather than a personality shaped by the beliefs and expectations of others. Authenticity rules!

## 3. Invest in at Least Eight High-Quality Relationships

I think that life is about connecting with people. For me, life is about loving them, laughing with them, learning from them, listening to them, being inspired by them, crying with them, encouraging them, following them, leading them through hard and good times, expressing feelings to them, being silent with them, and, most of all, helping them succeed and celebrating life with them.

But relationships can be complicated. Mine ended after ten years. Before I met Robbert, the longest relationship I had had lasted four years. I dated some men, and I loved to be wildly in love, but unconsciously I thought that the guys would not love me when they really got to know me. So after a few months I sabotaged everything, resulting in a breakup. The sad truth was that they did truly love me, but I did not love myself enough to accept that.

When I was diagnosed with MS, I had a conversation with a psychologist about how to cope with this chronic disease, and he wanted to study my personality. He asked me to imagine a line of little children. The children were all screaming because there was one piece of tasty candy and they all wanted to claim that piece, so they were yelling out loud: "It is for me! Give it to me! For me! Now!"

It was so noisy that you might not notice that there was one little girl, silently standing there, hopping from one leg to the other. She was shy and did not say one word as she watched the other kids fight for the candy. She didn't want the candy for herself; she wanted to give a piece to each of the other kids. That in itself would make her happy.

But it is a bit sad. Deep down she did not feel she deserved the candy for herself. That little girl was me, of course. When you relate that story to my overeating candy later in life, it all falls into place. The solution was for me to replace the candy with the belief that I deserved love.

Feeling worthy of love and happiness is your birthright. You don't have to change, you don't have to be fixed (because you are not broken), and you don't have to be cured. You are worthy of an abundance of love and happiness 24/7 for the rest of your life. The quality of your relationships will have a great impact on your feelings of happiness and love.

Goethe wrote, "The way you see people is the way you treat them and the way you treat them they will become."[2]

I think you should have at least eight high-quality friendships/relationships. How do you make sure that they are high quality? *Treat other people as if they are the most important person in your world, and*

2    Source: http://www.brainyquote.com/quotes/quotes/j/johannwolf378590.html.

*they will begin to treat you likewise.* I learned this important lesson from Brian Tracy. After all, everyone does the best they can, based on their past experiences and beliefs.

However, this can be easier said than done. Based what I've learned through counseling, study, and my own experiences, here are six practical ways to truly treat others well and develop high-quality relationships in your life:

**A. Believe that this person will totally exceed or meet your expectations and treat him or her that way.** My son, Daan, was having some tantrums as a result of the tension between his parents and of him being a two-year-old. In the beginning we would expect him to throw a tantrum or be negative, and of course he met that expectation. But when we changed our expectations of him and started to talk about him consistently as a happy, funny, big guy, he would glow with pride and start to act that way! So believe in others and treat them according to your beliefs. (Some people have low expectations or a lack of belief in themselves, so they will be suspicious in the beginning. Just persist and see what happens.)

**B. Give total support to what another is doing.** Help the person you're in relationship with succeed in what is important to him or her. I absolutely believe that one of the secrets to great relationships is helping others succeed in what is important to them—not what is important to you. Your partner will be so thankful if you offer your help.

**C. Try to understand the other person before you want the other person to understand you.** My ex had a tendency toward overly controlling behavior. Had I tried to understand the possible fear behind it, I could have reacted differently to his judging words. He, like any human, deserves all the love and happiness of the world; neither of us could give that, unfortunately. Sometimes people confuse showing control with showing love, and when you understand their fear behind it, it won't affect you that much anymore. Understanding is often better than just reacting.

So please step into the other's shoes before you state your opinion. Value the other person's opinion, too. As Stephen R. Covey said, first understand, then be understood.[3] Change your focus and see the situation from the other's perspective.

**D. When you are getting angry, simply wish the best for the other person.** However you feel toward this person, before even meet them or speak with this person, just wish the best for him or her. You will benefit greatly from this action. You can even say it out loud five times before interacting with the person. Your reaction will be milder than when you are driven by anger or frustration or other negative feelings. Wish this person the best in your heart and mind (even though it might not be congruent with your feelings) and watch what happens. We often blame our loved ones not because it helps, not because it is their fault, but because we feel better about ourselves by getting angry. Try not to blame.

To learn more, I highly recommend Brenda Soshanna's book *Fearless: 7 Principles of Peace of Mind*, (Sterling Ethos, 2012) and Brian Tracy's *Kiss that Frog: 12 Great Ways to Turn Negatives into Positives in Your Life and Work* (Berrett-Koehler Publishers, 2012).

**E. Be assertive, not aggressive or too quiet.** When you listen to someone's opinion, you are only listening—that does not mean you are agreeing with the opinion. Your partner or colleague can have a different opinion than yours; he or she has the right to have that. You can always share your own opinion as long as you can do it respectfully. Keep in mind to always be respectful, honest, and gentle. You can make this promise to yourself: I never want my partner, colleague, or

---

3    See Stephen R. Covey, *The 7 Habits of Highly Effective People* (Free Press, revised 2004).

friend to feel sad or bad when we don't agree, and it is okay when we don't agree.

Be careful with words. Use the words "I love you *and* . . ." instead of "I love you *but* . . ."

**F. Do not assume you know everything.** It is possible that you don't know everything you need to know until you ask! The way you ask and when you ask are important, of course. This is what my psychotherapist friend taught me: start by asking for an appointment. "We have challenges, so shall we schedule a time for us to talk about how we can meet them?" Ask a lot of questions and listen carefully.

> ♥   Do you think you need to improve your relationships?
> ♥   Which of the items above speak to you?
> I sincerely hope you will try one or two of them in the coming weeks and see if they help you.

## 4. Ignite More Passion in Your Life

Passion is the fuel of the heart. Passion is the powerful combination of enthusiasm and energy and love. Passion is the magic force that pulls us forward effortlessly. When we are filled with passion, we don't need to push ourselves forward with the help of external rewards like money or applause. When you are passionate, whether it is about your life, your work, yourself, or your partner, you are on fire. But you have to ignite it within yourself before you can experience it in something else.

To create more passion in your life, focus on doing those things that make you forget the time, that generate energy in you, that make your eyes shine brightly. You probably know what you are passionate about, but are you living and expressing your passion on a daily or even a weekly basis?

> When you are feeling happy, engaged, and connected with yourself, what are you doing?

If you show up daily with enough energy and enthusiasm, you will be amazed by the change in people's reaction to you. If you can share your passion, it becomes contagious and people will be more than eager to help you fulfill your dreams.

Energy and enthusiasm are things you can decide to amplify in your life. You don't need to find them first; you can decide to be more energetic and enthusiastic and passionate while you go through your day. Be prepared for love. Just give everything and hold nothing back, participate 100 percent, and you will feel so alive. Give all that you are to your life, and enjoy each moment. Never forget to notice all the miracles that happen in each moment. Don't take everything for granted. The love of your partner or friend or kids is not less magical because it will be still there tomorrow and the day after that.

How passionate you are in life is a good indicator of how happy you are in your life, and the moment you start incorporating more passion and more enthusiasm into your day, the sooner you will notice that the habits your unhappy self has developed (such as overeating) tend to retreat in the wake of that passion.

If your heart is singing because of all the passion flooding through it, if you are busy with something in which you can express your passion and love, the urge to go to the store to buy a candy bar will decrease, instantly. Passion and mindless overeating are not a good team.

On a higher level, if you can find something that you love to do and that can help other people, you will be rewarded abundantly with love and gratefulness, and, again, you will be less likely to turn to food to feel better.

Now ignite that smoldering passion inside of you again and let it burn brightly, and it might even light the way for other people, too.

### 5. Make Three Expressions of Gratitude on a Daily Basis

On Valentine's Day, 2011, I saw a video of motivational speaker/coach Tony Robbins for the first time. Robbert, my ex-husband, asked me to watch it because Tony was talking about the company Robbert worked for at that time. I saw a big guy sitting next to a blond lady in a golf cart, and I was intrigued. I decided to visit his website, and, some weeks later, I bought a program about how to create a business online.

My weight management institute was getting a bit too much to handle, and I was looking for ways to share my knowledge in another way. Unfortunately, my MS relapsed and I needed to go to the hospital for treatment. I had my laptop with me and the DVDs from Tony Robbins. I was in a ward with three other people with severe neurological problems, and they smelled because they were incontinent. One of them had MS in a severe progressive state.

The environment could have depressed me, reminding me of my possible future, but learning new skills gave me hope for a better future—and I love learning. The nurses even asked me if Tony was my husband, seeing me laughing out loud behind my laptop, with an IV in my arm. Unfortunately I got a rare anaphylactic allergic reaction because of the medicine, resulting in the ceasing of the treatment. My heart rate dropped to 50, and with a blood pressure of 90/50, I barely escaped death.

The doctors decided that simple bedrest was the best treatment for me. They did not want to try any new medicine.

When I got home, I felt grateful for having learned so many new things, because it gave me the power and the excitement to be able to create a new future. It gave me new perspective. So I decided I should buy something for Tony and two other mentors to show them my gratitude.

If I had been in the hospital with a different mindset, I could have complained a lot about the fact that there were smelly and often dribbling people around me, that the treatment was for nothing (and the side effects like acne and weight gain were terrible), that I would never be cured from relapse since my heart rate dropped with the medication, and so on. But that is not who I am. I will always look for opportunities in bad situations to improve them or make them more bearable. And I am always grateful: for my life, which I've almost lost a few times now; for my kids; for my parents; for my house; for my friends, all of them; and for my mentors in life—and that includes my ex-husband.

And you know what? Creatively showing your gratitude to others is more fulfilling than eating candy or cake. It makes you happy, and it makes the receiver happy. And happiness is contagious.

I think it is important to show people how grateful you are for what they are doing for you or just for who they are. It makes me happy. Be generous with your compliments and little gifts. It has brought me so many magic moments with people. It makes life abundant instead of deprived, no matter how much or how little money we have or how many challenges we face.

Being grateful allows you to act from a place of abundance instead of feeling deprived. You can elevate your happiness ten times if you learn to be so grateful for what you have, what you learn, who you meet, and where you are in your life. Compare yourself to who you were yesterday or last year instead of comparing yourself to more successful or happier people. Be grateful that you have a healthy body that you will take care of from now on. Be grateful for all the little things in life, and you will be more happy and less prone to overeating. Be thankful for your fears, because they reveal your opportunities for growth in life. You even can be grateful for all your mistakes because they allowed you to improve yourself.

For example, I can be grateful for my divorce because I had to learn to be completely independent, and that was a huge opportunity for growth in my life. Of course, I am grateful for the positive things too, for all the smiles and hugs and kisses I received; for all the love, especially the precious love from my kids; for the help and love from my parents; for the laughter and friendship and the nice experiences with my friends—I love all that. When I look out my window and see the beautiful landscape, I am so grateful for the place I live, and when I learn new things from my mentors I am so grateful to have them in my life.

You have at least fifty things to be very grateful for. Write them down in your journal and make it a habit from now on to note at least three things that you are grateful for on a daily basis.

---

- ♥ What are you grateful for in your life?
- ♥ Who deserves a big thank-you from you, expressed in a creative way?
- ♥ What can you thank yourself for?
- ♥ Are you grateful for all the love in your life? You will notice that the more grateful you are for love in your life, the more abundantly it will come to you!
- ♥ Can you try to be grateful for your problems, viewing them as opportunities for you to learn and grow?
- ♥ Are you grateful for your body, which still functions after you have not been treating it with care and love?
- ♥ Every time before you go to sleep, think of or write down three things that made you grateful.

## 6. Let Go of the Past

When I was a child, I adored Minet, my older sister's doll. She had long brown and green hair and spots of red nail polish on her lips, and she had a rock-hard body. No, she was not the most beautiful doll. In fact, she was quite ugly. She was not soft at all or advanced in any way. But my love for her made her very soft and beautiful. In my five-year-old eyes, she was the prettiest and most gentle doll on earth, and I took care of her like she was a real baby.

But sometimes I had enough of her and I threw her in the corner. Or under my bed. With strength. Eventually I exchanged her for another doll. That other doll had short black hair. Unfortunately, that sweet doll and I did not get along. Not at all. I tried to love her, but it did not work. There was no magic between us. The poor little doll never got a name. Secretly I dreamed of a real baby doll, but my mother said that was too expensive. Years and years later, when my sister's daughter reached the age when she began to play with dolls, I instantly bought her a baby doll—a real one, soft, with pink clothes and pretty blue eyes.

As wonderful as new toys are, giving a wrapped gift to a child can sometimes be frustrating for her, because the object of her desire is securely tied up in its packaging, with layers of paper and cellophane tape. All the magnificent accessories are hard to get to, and sometimes she gets hurt when she tries to detach the toy from the packaging. After a lot of wrangling, she can finally get her hands on the shiny toy and actually play with it.

If you want to give *yourself* a real gift, "unwrap" or detach yourself from the past. Get rid of the packaging and paper and tape that still tie you to the past. Only then will you be able to enjoy your present. Untying the ropes that secure you to the past is not the same as cutting all the strings. You don't need to forget or deny your past; you just won't be controlled by it anymore. Fully detaching yourself means that you give yourself permission to be free instead of being a marionette, living a life that is restricted by invisible cords, tied to your past.

It is time now to untie these cords and cut these strings. Although it might hurt, it gives you space to focus on the present and create your healthier and happier future. Transform yourself from a victim of the past to the producer of your ideal future.

The fact is that what has happened in the past cannot be changed anymore, and it has made you the magnificent person you are today. Your experiences from the past might help others to progress when you tell them about your struggles and success, but don't let those past experiences determine your future. If you can shine a different light on those experiences, they won't cast a large shadow over the rest of your life. Untie all the cords so you can play fully in the present moment.

The well-known author Dr. Wayne Dyer says that it is never too late to have a happy childhood. You can choose to see your childhood in a new way.

"What's past is prologue," wrote Shakespeare in his play *The Tempest*. Everything that happened to you in the past has been a preparation for you becoming a better you and preparing for your magnificent life ahead.

I would love to write a little bit about forgiveness, because becoming free in this moment has a lot to do with forgiving the past.

We all have experienced bad things done to us by someone else. Even if they happened years and years ago, we may still feel bitterness and resentment.

I know you will say, "But, Pauline, you have no idea what he or she did to me! It is unforgivable!" And you are right; I have no idea and I am sorry for you. But the bitterness of holding on to that old pain is far more harmful to your heart than you can imagine. When you forgive someone else, it does not mean that you accept or allow that behavior. It means that you allow yourself to be free and that you are no longer trying to get even. Getting even means getting bitter (because you will eventually get back what you give). Forgiving means freedom. It means that you are no longer willing to allow that experience to harmfully affect your life.

Lift your self-worth to a level where you accept only loving experiences in your life, please. And stop putting up with things you know you should not tolerate for one second more. It all has to do with self-esteem and self-love. When you know that you are worthy of being free and not being held hostage by your anger, it is easier to forgive. When you stay angry with someone, you continue to feel victimized, and thus you lose an incredible amount of energy in blaming—and blaming keeps you caught in the problem! Regain your energy, your power, and your self-esteem by learning to forgive.

People do the best they can with the awareness, skills, character, and understanding that they have. If they hurt you, they probably have been hurt too, maybe as a child. Try to look with compassionate eyes and do what you can to set yourself free. Write a letter (you don't need to post it), make a phone call, schedule an appointment, or just write it all down and burn the paper. Make a ritual. Don't accept the bad behavior or make excuses for it. It has nothing to do with the one who mistreated you. It has to do with you deciding to get out of the dark prison of the past. It is your time to dance in the sunlight of life again.

♥ Untie yourself from the past
♥ Forgive and let go
♥ Be present

When you finally have removed that emotional clutter, it is a good idea to clean the excess clutter in your house too, allowing all the positive energy and creativity back in your environment. With good music on and an open window, sort your stuff out. Use a throw away box, a charity box, and a keep box. You will feel so much lighter after doing this! Throw away your "fat" clothes, too—you will not need them anymore. Put objects in your house that make you feel good, like fresh flowers or pictures, and put on music that you love. When you eat alone, make the table look as if you were expecting a guest. It is important that you take better care not only of your body but of your daily environment, too.

### 7. Season the Dough of Your Heart with a Daily Shot of Positivity and Inspiration

I strongly believe in the power of positivity and inspiration in your daily environment.

> ♥ Surround yourself with positive, supporting people.
>
> ♥ Surround yourself with art that touches your soul.
>
> ♥ Surround yourself with pictures of people whom you love.
>
> ♥ Surround yourself with flowers, candles, music—whatever makes you feel good.
>
> ♥ Surround yourself with cushions and blankets that make you feel comfortable.
>
> ♥ Make your workplace beautiful and inspiring, with fresh flowers, photos, or quotes that you love.
>
> ♥ Make your bathroom look like a spa, just by adding some candles and waxing lights to it.
>
> ♥ Create more magic moments with people by being present with them.

When my parents came to my house during the time of my divorce, the energy shifted immediately. It was more positive, lighter, and sweeter, and a warm blanket of gratitude, pride, and an abundance of love filled the house, removing the heavy atmosphere of a broken marriage that resulted in angry and sad hearts. My parents injected the house with an antidote that made all of us happy again.

My mother laughs out loud, and it feels fresh in the house. The children are so happy that they dance for my parents. Kiki is wearing her princess dress, and she dances with her father to Pachelbel's wedding march. Daan is jumping between them, and sometimes he bends forward, standing on his hands, and he lifts his right leg in the air. He bows afterward, waiting for applause. He then suddenly mistakes the music for our national anthem, so he stands straight up with his little two-year-old hand on his heart, and he looks like he is the king of the Netherlands. The children bow several times, and we applaud for them.

My parents are filled with pride and joy; I am touched by what I witness and feel a bit sad, seeing my ex-husband doing his best to make this day a good day. He makes us a delicious spinach meal.

Those moments happen often in life, even when the times are rough, and you should create more of them. They can take place only when you are present enough to really enjoy the moment. *Never focus too much on your problems while there is still so much to laugh about and so many to love.*

Magic moments give life that extra glow, and they make your heart sing instead of cry.

After a magic moment, you will feel better about yourself and others than you did before the moment. You will experience more love or more pride or more intimacy or more fun. You are enjoying your life in this moment with passion, and you are not worrying about the past or the future. Always be present in the moment.

Being present in the moment includes sometimes taking a break from looking at displays. I highly recommend one display diet a week: no iPod, iPad, iPhone, laptop computer, or TV screen.

My grandfather lived his whole life without any of these things, and he was very happy. He has been my inspiration for my entire life, and you can read more about his story in chapter 5. He made me want to be a better person, just like my father inspired me to create a better future, my kids inspire me daily to leave a great legacy, and you, the reader, inspired me to write this book, to give it my best so it serves you. I am not inspired by playing Angry Birds or spending time on Facebook. It distracts me. Your life deserves a display diet too, one day every week.

When you are near the end of your life, sitting in your rocking chair, you won't remember TV shows. You will remember the happy times you spent with your friends and loved ones and the victories you had. Think about that when you resist turning off your TV. Do you really think that you will be proud of yourself when you look back and remember that you never missed an episode of *Seinfeld*, but forgot to express your gratitude to your friends and family? That you always enjoyed *The Voice*, but never dared to share your own voice with the world because you stopped learning and improving yourself?

Positivity and inspiration are the best tastemakers for life. When you feel positive and inspired, you live with gusto. So take some action to feel positive and inspired!

# Chapter 2

# GROW YOUR BRAIN AND
# UPGRADE YOUR THINKING

*Life consists in what a man is thinking of all day.*
— Ralph Waldo Emerson

Size matters. I am not referring to your waist size or to the size of your clothes. Or anything else.

The bigger your brain, the bigger your capacity to think, to make better decisions, and to act better. Better decisions lead to better results; better results lead to more happiness in life; more happiness makes it easier to live a healthy life. Your brain is the source of all your actions, your decisions, your beliefs, your dreams, your inspiration, and your imagination.

Daniel Amen, MD, a famous brain expert who spoke at Brendon Burchard's High Performance Academy, says that brains shrink when you are overweight or obese. This effect is called the Dinosaur Syndrome: the bigger the belly, the smaller the brain—and extinction threatens. When I heard that I was intrigued—and a bit frightened.

But the solution to the Dinosaur Syndrome is profound and simple: Turn fat into love.

Dinosaur Syndrome: big belly, small brain, and extinction.

Turning Fat into Love: big heart, big brain, small belly, and expansion of love for life.

Your brain should, like your heart, grow to size XXL, as soon as possible. Neuroscientists call the changeable quality of the brain *neuroplasticity*.

In this chapter I will discuss five steps that will help you to think better and be smarter and more positive, so you can make better decisions and get results that propel you forward. You will be able to make decisions that will help you create more of the life you dream of.

> Do you refresh your browser on your computer often? Do you update your programs when necessary? Your brain might still run outdated and old programs, just as a computer can. Upgrading your thinking and growing your brain will help you a lot!

Here are the most important rules for upgrading your thinking, followed by an effective plan that will grow your brain.

## 1. Own Your Fat

*You cannot change the circumstances, the seasons,*
*or the wind, but you can change yourself.*
—Jim Rohn

"What is the use of education when I have no future? I have quit university already." In the hospital bed in front of me sat a young girl of twenty-three, with an IV in her arm like me, getting Prednisolon treatments for a relapse of MS.

"You what?!" I could not believe what I was hearing.

"I left the university. I had two more years to go, but I saw no reason to finish it after I got diagnosed with MS." I could not hide my disapproval. She looked at me as if I had no brains in my head. And then she started to convince me in every way possible that creating a better future for herself was useless.

The terrible MS was to blame for everything that was going wrong in her life. She had decided not to move in with her boyfriend because she doubted whether she would be able to stay in a relationship with him—she was often too tired to do fun stuff and she had too much pain in her body to be friendly to him. She had also already decided to give up on becoming a mother.

After listening to her for ten minutes, I interrupted her endless complaining by getting out of my bed and pulling up a chair next to her bed. "Stop," I said as boldly as I could. "Listen to me, please. I recognize your feelings because I have been there, too. I know that it is overwhelming, especially the uncertainty of your future. It is terrifying. MS can feel like your thinking is covered with a thick layer of fog in your head. But never, ever give your power away to your disease. No matter what, you have MS, but you are not MS."

She looked very angry, but I was determined to make my point, and continued. "I have been at that crossroads too, but I decided to live from hope, not from fear. And yes, life will sometimes be more difficult for you than for your healthy friends, but this disease is your opportunity to expand or to shrink. You won't see it now, but you have got to have faith in yourself and your future."

She replied that she did not want to grow and that she did not want to have faith, and I realized that she felt so comfortable playing the victim that she would not easily give up that role. I had the suspicion that she had done that long before the diagnosis.

I told her my story of struggle and my refusal to give up on my dreams. Ever. I told her that after my diagnosis I had lived in New Zealand, had graduated, had married, and had started my own company. And then I showed her a picture of my two beautiful little kids. Tears started rolling down her face, and she said very softly, "You are a mother!" At that moment her boyfriend walked in and, seeing her tears, started to cry as well. I felt a bit awkward and left them alone, my IV pole hampering my attempt at a graceful exit.

Later he came back to me and thanked me for giving them a different perspective, and with a big smile they both walked away, breathing hope and love into their future. I have never seen that girl again, but I think and hope she has followed her dreams instead of her fears.

Never give your power away to things that you cannot control. Stay responsible for creating the life that you desire and deserve. You are responsible for everything in your life. Every time you blame someone else for your big belly, every time you blame the rain that you cannot exercise, every time it is your mother-in-law's fault that you ate the cake, you will shrink a little inside and probably grow a little on the outside. You will turn love into fat, because you have given your power away!

It is time to turn that around: Let your inner self grow and become so in balance that you only make decisions that are congruent with you becoming happier and healthier. If your decisions are not moving you forward, they are not the right decisions. Choose to create those experiences that are most supportive in your quest for more health and happiness and love. It is totally up to you. Nobody is responsible for your health or your happiness. You are in total control. That might be hard to accept, because we easily blame others for bad stuff that happens in our lives, but we are always in total control about how we react to those bad events.

Imagine what freedom you will feel when you are the only one responsible for your life. That means that you no longer need to change somebody else, you no longer need to blame somebody else when things go wrong, you no longer need to procrastinate or cancel exercising because of something or somebody else. You need to change you. If you are unhappy, it is your responsibility to change that. No one else but you can make you change inside. Stop looking outside yourself to explain why you are not yet the most happy and healthy person in the world. Be a victor, not a victim. Don't become like the girl in the hospital, blaming and complaining and feeling even more miserable. You either contributed to how your life is right now, or you just let it happen. When you want change, you need to accept the fact that you are the only one responsible for having created your results, and that you are the one who can change everything.

It is time that your appearance becomes more congruent with your shining self. Grow inside and lose weight outside.

You can create progress and success only if you accept that you are responsible for the results you have in your life. Not anyone or anything else. You.

Here are three action steps for taking 100 percent responsibility:

1.  Refuse to blame anything or anyone.
2.  Accept no excuses for not making progress toward your happier and healthier future on a daily basis.
3.  Find an accountability partner to help you stay on track, preferably someone who likes physical exercise more than you do.

## 2. Don't Talk about Fat, but Give Your Dreams a Voice

*Be clear in your own mind exactly what you are after.*
—Benjamin Franklin

This is a little story from Idries Shah: A man had a bowl of very sour pickles, and he ate one after the other. Every time he took a bite from a new pickle, it tasted so sour that tears ran from his eyes and his face made awful grimaces. His friend watched him and asked, "Why do you continue eating those sour pickles?" The man replied, "Because I am hoping for a sweet one."

We have all been there. We all eat sour pickles, wishing they will turn into sweet ones.

With tears in our eyes and a disgusting taste in our mouth, we try to change the things we don't want into the things we want more of. Fear into more confidence. Exhaustion into more energy. Fat into more health. Unattractiveness into more beauty. Deprivation into more abundance. Chaos into more harmony.

We talk about our problems, we think about our problems, we listen to our problems—and guess what happens? We live our problems, or, if not, we almost become our problems. The solution is both simple and profound.

Shift your entire focus to the things you do want instead of the things you don't want. Talk about the things you do want. Think about the things you do want. Dream about the things you do want. See the things you do want clearly in your head. Meditate about the things you do want. Write about the things you do want. Set goals to achieve the things you do want.

And then, of course, *take action*, every day.

Some examples of eating sour pickles we probably all can relate to:

- Trying to change somebody but not succeeding.
- Wishing to see someone new/better/smarter/younger/ prettier in our mirror, but stubbornly refusing to love, trust, and believe in ourselves every time we look in that same mirror.
- Hoping we will be happier when the chocolate goes into the mouth, but feeling even worse afterward.
- Blaming anybody else for our problems, but feeling extremely powerless after doing so.

You need to have it very clear in your mind where you want to go, who you want to become, and what is needed to get there. Anything else will only waste your time, your energy, your health, and, yes, even your love.

You waste time, because even if you had twenty-five hours a day, if you give your power away to the wrong things and blame other people, you will never create any of the results you deserve.

You waste your energy, because you will feel more tired instead of alive, because you are not plugged in to your own power plant, but instead are leaking energy to others.

You waste your health, because your body will ask for soothing things like sweet comfort food to be consoled by you when you are thinking about your future in a negative way. Your body will give you excuses for not living healthily because you are not thinking that your health truly matters, and thus that your life doesn't truly matter. But it does matter.

And you waste love, because you fill your heart with fear and negativity and feelings of deprivation, instead of coming from a place of abundance, love, and faith.

Of course, fear will always exist, negative experiences will occur, and negative people will exist. That is part of life.

But you should ask yourself if you are going to continue to eat from a bowl of sour pickles, hoping they turn sweet, or make the effort required to create a bowl full of sweet pickles? Here are some questions to consider:

1. Before you began reading this book, what were you focused on? Were you talking and thinking about your problems and worries? Or were you turning dreams into reality by speaking and thinking about them and taking action to make them real?
2. What are you going to put your focus on from now on? What is the first step?
3. What do you want more of?
4. Who do you need to become so that you can turn your dreams into reality?

## 3. Ready, Steady . . . Stuck

You might have heard this story before from Les Brown, a famous motivational speaker, but I like it so much that I share it again here.

A man walked past a house and saw on the porch an old lady rocking in her chair and a dog lying next to her, moaning as if he were in a lot of pain. As the man passed, he wondered what the dog was moaning about. The next day, he walked again past the house, and the dog was still moaning. The man could not resist asking, "Excuse me, lady. What is wrong with your dog?"

"Oh, him?" she said. "He is just lying on a nail."

"But why doesn't he get up, then?" the man replied, confused by her answer.

The old lady smiled and said, "Well, it hurts enough for him to moan about it, but not enough for him to move yet."

I love that story because it is so true. When we are lying on a nail it hurts, and we are moaning but not moving. As I said earlier, talking about our problems with others or in our head should not be confused with taking action.

Talking takes your time; progress takes your action. And talking action is not the same as taking action. Taking new actions will give new results and new outcomes. We are not guaranteed to have great outcomes, so we might ask ourselves, "But what if I fail?"

Let me ask you: What *if* you fail? Would that be the end of the world? Or just a lesson learned? What if it turns out great?

You should ask yourself every day, in every situation: How is it going to be better than this? How am I going to get there? What is my next step? What should I be doing right now?

You may have heard of the book *The Secret*; you may have even read it. I believe that the writers of that book accidentally forgot to mention the real secret. The real secret to more happiness, success, and health was left out.

You can wish, you can visualize, you can create vision boards, you can dream, and you can meditate, but you will find yourself in the same place as you are now, one year, two years, or even twenty-five years from now, if you refuse to get off your nail.

If you don't take the risk, if you don't take any action, you will be repeating the same story over and over again.

So if that is the secret to success, why aren't we all staggeringly successful? What keeps us from taking action?

Taking new action forces us to feel uncomfortable, to get off the couch, to stretch our boundaries, to get behind our fears, to move through our obstacles, to develop new skills, to face dreamkillers.

Not taking any action is so much easier! We can just press the Repeat button of our past behaviors, and we will get the same results over and over.

I am here to tell you to push the Pause button for a while. Slow down before you speed up. Pause now. Be silent. Remind yourself of your why. Remind yourself what it would mean for others if you finally decide to step up and become the most happy and healthy person you can be.

And know that you will be uncomfortable for a while, until your new lifestyle becomes a habit. It will be uncomfortable for two to three weeks.

When you start seeing taking new action as *practice*, everything shifts. Everything. Practice means that you can fail several times before you succeed. Practice means that you need to repeat it several times before you master it. Practice means that it is never a failure when you don't get the immediate results you had hoped for.

> *There is only one thing that makes a dream*
> *impossible to achieve: the fear of failure.*
> —Paulo Coelho

Real failure is the refusal to learn the lessons from your past mistakes, and you will repeat those mistakes until you get the lesson. Adopt a mindset of learning the lessons in joy and peace, instead of trying to learn from fear or pain or deprivation. Life is full of lessons that are necessary for us to grow and blossom, and if we refuse to learn them the lesson will be presented over and over again!

Not everything has to be perfect at once. Fail forward, but you must try first before you quit.

For weight loss this is extremely important. Take action toward your healthier self and be committed.

No new action means no progress. Please do not compare yourself to others, but to who you were yesterday.

How do you start to outperform yourself on a daily basis? How do you start to change?

**1. Raise the bar for what you expect for yourself in life, not making excuses, not accepting less than the highest quality of your efforts, and expecting the best result.** Expect the best results from taking action, although it is practice. You don't get in life what you want, but what you expect. So expect the best. Make that a mantra. Expect the best. I don't mean that everything in your life should be or ever will be perfect. But you should always expect the best of every situation, no matter what the result will be. Have faith that you can handle whatever outcome will occur. You expect the best, and you can handle it.

**2. Accept discomfort, fear, and failure at the same time.** Welcome those feelings instead of fighting them. Welcome them, feel them, and release them. You will have to pay the price now for the reward later. Please be willing to be very, very uncomfortable and probably even scared for a while. This is the only way to victory. This is the only way to change. This is the way out of your current situation and toward the better destination you deserve.

**3. Become aware and change the words you use** (see the Don't Talk Fat section in chapter 2). Turn "can't" into "can," "probably" into "certainly." Problems are possibilities to grow. Exercise is a treatment instead of a punishment. Tired is a chance to level up your energy or to go to sleep. Be aware of old stories and excuses that have sabotaged your progress for long enough now. Stories can change, and if you change your story, you change yourself.

**4. Find cheerleaders who will support you, motivate you, and hold you accountable.** This is so important. You should surround yourself with at least three people who will help you and lift you up.

**5. Establish deadlines and rewards to help you to stay on track.** You can lose an average of two pounds a week. Reward yourself for every ten pounds of weight loss with a spa treatment or a night out with a friend. You might want to walk daily for ninety minutes effortlessly within three months, and you should reward yourself when you accomplish that goal. Take your calendar, mark some deadlines, communicate them with your cheerleaders and accountability partner, and be creative in your reward for yourself. Having goals and deadlines is important, although you should never stress about a number on the scale. In fact, I suggest you put the scale away if you have a tendency to stand on it every day.

## 4. Turn on the Light

When two-year-old Daan has a nightmare about crocodiles or owls, I turn on the light and show him that everything is safe. He is reassured enough that he is back to sleep again within two minutes.

When we have limiting beliefs about ourselves or unrealistic fears, it is not easy to turn on the light to reassure ourselves that it was only a bad dream.

Although I have a disease that has the potential to paralyze my body, it was I who paralyzed my life by believing the fears in my heart and the thoughts in my head of not being good enough. I was stuck and overweight, and I could not make any movement in my life. But I felt so much lighter after I released excess emotional weight that I started to fly effortlessly and created more of the life and the healthier body that I deserved. I let go of my fears by finally realizing that I was held hostage by them, and suddenly I found out that the door of this self-created prison was open and had been open all the time. I thought this door could be opened only by external praise, external love, or external rewards like food or money. But this has never been necessary, because this door was open all the time.

I stepped through this door too, leaving behind the darkness of fear, the shadows of doubt, and the heavy weight of a small self-esteem. It was as if I, like Daan, woke up from having a bad dream and realized that it was only a dream. The antidote to these fears, again, was not eating them away, not seeking love to melt them, and not letting others praise me so they would disappear. It was simply connecting to my own internal power, feeling my fears, looking them in the eye, and taking action anyway, no matter how scared I was. *Whoosh*, they were gone. (I highly recommend Susan Jeffers' book *Feel the Fear and Do it Anyway*, Fawcett, 1987.)

Fear of failure is like the crocodile under Daan's bed: just an illusion, not based on any truth.

It feels real, but it is only a little part of our mind telling you that you can't and you should not. But when you turn on the light in your whole mind, when you see clearly with your whole mind, doubts and fears become transparent. They are just a part of your ego mind that causes you trouble, but you are so much more than that. When you are able to see with your whole mind and heart, you don't judge or paralyze yourself; you love. That is why I think we should supersize our heart and grow our brain. Connect with the wholeness of your mind, not just the ego part that keeps you small. Connect with the light coming from your heart, let it flow through your body, and let it put a spotlight on who you are becoming. Have faith.

Sometimes you don't think you have any fears, but you still feel stuck. What is happening then? Your subconscious can cause you to think and behave in a way that you did not intend. You create the wrong results or unconsciously stop creating good results because something in the basement of your mind is sabotaging all your efforts.

It is important for me to share this with you, because you might have thoughts or beliefs in your unconscious mind that can block your progress. The language of the subconscious is not English or Dutch or Italian, but it speaks in images and colors and music. In that way you can talk to and access this basement of your mind, this subconscious mind, where balloons of fears and doubts (often placed there in your childhood) are floating around. It is time that you release some of those bubbles into the sky. If you release some of your balloons, others may come up, so it is a constant process of releasing and being with the feelings you want to avoid or eat away.

Here is an exercise I did with my clients.

Imagine yourself blowing air into a black balloon, and every breath you blow into that balloon stands for every fear, every excuse, every thought of not being good enough that has been holding you back for too long now. Each time you breathe in, think of the word "love." Each time you breathe out into the balloon, think of a phrase to represent those things that are holding you back: "fear of rejection," "fear of failure," and so on. Use the words that feel the strongest for you.

You might have to blow five balloons to catch all your fears. Or ten.

Blow into the balloons all your fears, excuses, and limiting beliefs.

And then imagine letting them go out of your head, like helium balloons flying into the sky toward the sun, transforming from heavy black balloons into transparent light and thin air.

There is more space in you now after releasing all these fears and doubts. You are lighter now. You have released excess weight.

## 5. Your Big Brain Plan

When we start to use our whole mind, we should take excellent care of it, too. Having a brain disease myself, I have learned some tricks and tips that helped me grow my brain and keep it in great shape.

Here is my Big Brain Plan in a nutshell.

### Take a Vitamin D Supplement

A lot of people have a shortage of vitamin D without knowing it. It is good for your brain and for your skin and bones. We are using more sunscreen (and we should continue to do that!) and we are indoors more than we are outdoors, so we are not getting enough vitamin D from the sun. You should have your vitamin D level checked and get advice from a medical practitioner on the amount you need for optimal health.

### Take a Fish Oil Supplement That Contains Vitamin E

Fish oil combines beauty with brains. Fish oil is the best wonder pill I know of; it takes care of your heart, brain, skin, and mood at the same time. It has mood-stabilizing properties, it lowers triglyceride levels, and it has immune system–enhancing and nerve cell–stabilizing properties. It even acts as an anti-inflammatory. I give my kids fish oil every day. You should take it every day, too. Use only the highly purified types, free of PCBs and mercury. I invest in more expensive fish oil so that I know I don't buy contaminated oil. Most people are deficient in this important omega-3 fat but have too much omega-6 fat. If you are allergic to fish oil, try plant-derived DHA, made from microalgae.

### Eat Low-Calorie Foods That Are High in Antioxidants

Foods that are healthy for your body and heart are healthy for your brain as well. Here are some good foods that are high in antioxidants: blueberries, blackberries, strawberries, oranges, prunes, Brussel sprouts, avocados, kiwis, broccoli, and spinach.

### Eliminate Caffeine; Drink Water or Green Tea

Caffeine restricts the blood flow to your brain and causes you to have more belly fat. You should drink a lot more water or green tea instead! Make it a habit to have bottles of water with you everywhere you go. You will not only think better, but you will also look younger and fresher. Beautiful skin means a beautiful brain.

### Stop Eating Sugar

Sugar gives you empty calories and bad teeth and has no nutritional value. Stop adding sugar to tea or coffee, stop drinking soft drinks, and decrease the amount of cookies and cakes and candy you consume drastically, to just once a month or once every two weeks.

### Relax and Take It Easy!

Relaxing is so vital for your brain. Meditate, read, or take a bath, and sleep when you are tired. Learn to say no so you can say yes more often to yourself.

### Exercise Your Brain

### Physical Exercise

What is good for your body and heart is good for your brain, too. Because you increase the blood flow to the brain and it lowers your stress level, try to do intensive aerobic exercise three times per week. If you hate the gym, there are alternatives.

What physical activity did you like to do when you were a kid? Biking, hula-hooping, roller skating? You don't need to go to the gym to do exercise! Do what you like. Work to an intensity such that you can still talk but not sing.

*Learn*

The brain is capable of making new connections. When you learn new things, your brain will make new connections! So learn a new language, read books, go to a class—it's good for your brain! Don't take the same route to your work every day; get off your autopilot.

*Listen to Classical Music*

The first year of my daughter's life, she heard classical music every day before she went to sleep. She slept like a baby, and she is very intelligent and balanced. I give credit to the fish oil and the classical music to which she was exposed as her brain developed.

You can download a PDF with an extended list of healthy brain food for free at www.turningfatintolove.com. Go online and do that!

# Chapter 3

# HIGH FIVE TO IMPROVE YOUR LIFE

N ow that we have supersized our heart and grown our brain, it is time to think about our body.

I am sure you have changed your life or lost weight before; this probably isn't your first journey toward more health and happiness. Perhaps you even thought you had reached your destination, but the change did not last. To create long-term results for the rest of your life, you need to prepare yourself in a way you may not have prepared yourself before.

The following five items will get you prepared: they will help you find motivation from within, stay on track and make progress, and get back up after a setback. I call them the High Five to Improve Your Life, because they have a high impact on your *long-term* physical and mental transformation.

## 1. Picture Your Dream Future—and your Nightmare Future

I think it is important to get crystal clear on what direction you are choosing in your life. At this moment, you have come to a crossroads, and you can commit to becoming your best self or you can commit to your old habits: the choice is up to you.

Let's say we could put you in a time machine and show you two previews of your future ten years from now. The first preview shows you hanging out with your friends on Thanksgiving Day—laughing, talking, and having fun. You seem to be very happy and you see yourself smile a lot. Your face looks older, you have more grey hair, but it is you. But then the camera zooms in to your shoes. And you notice that although it is winter time, you are wearing flipflops. You don't understand why—it can't be that your belly is preventing you from putting on your own shoes, can it? No, that would be impossible . . . But the clothes you wear don't reflect your taste, or any fashion at all; these are just sacks . . . And when you look more closely at your face, you see that your chin has almost disappeared! You see fat everywhere on your body, and when you look into your own eyes, you see that you are not genuinely happy with yourself, and that you try to cover that up with laughing so much. While you are watching this preview, you feel both disgusted about yourself and sorry for yourself, and you cannot believe you did not made the decision to change.

The second preview also shows you ten years from now, and you watch yourself hanging out with your friend on Thanksgiving Day, laughing, talking, and having fun. You are the host, and you manage everything very well. As you walk around, you look beautiful, fit, and very confident, and you wear clothes that suit you. When you look more closely at your face, you see that your skin is glowing, you have a healthy blush in your cheeks, and although you have grey hair, you look almost younger than you do today! While you are watching this preview, you feel so proud of yourself. At the end of the preview you see yourself dance—you dance as if nobody is watching, but everybody is watching. Everybody is watching you being you, fully expressed, fully confident and fullfilled. Everybody enjoys your dancing, including you. As you watch, you try to remember the last time you danced so freely and so confidently. You feel so proud of the person you have chosen to become, and almost a bit jealous of that happy and healthy person, the one who you truly are meant to be.

He or she is already inside you, dear reader. Your future whispers to you, and which scenario you choose is up to you. Which one do *you* choose?

We all inherently gain weight as we age; unfortunately we don't have to eat anything more or move any less for that to happen. Add bad food habits and less exercise to this process, and you can imagine that future you with a big belly is not that far from the truth. But you can reverse all of that: you can change the direction; you are able to make the shift.

---

What would you do differently if your body was 100 percent fit and slim, and you had an abundance of energy every moment?

♥ Would you feel differently?

♥ Speak differently?

♥ Think differently?

♥ Would you feel more confident?

- ♥ How would you feel and think if you were fifty pounds heavier than you are now?
- ♥ How would it affect your work?
- ♥ Your relationships?
- ♥ Your self-esteem?
- ♥ Your self-image?
- ♥ And how would it affect your health?
- ♥ Would you be ill? Would you have developed type 2 diabetes?

## 2. Plan Your Workouts, Exercise, and Me Time

Mary Kay Ash said, "Plan your work and work your plan."

If you have decided to pursue your dream future rather than waiting for your nightmare future, it is time to plan.

From now on you must plan what is important to you. Many of us excel at taking care of others or doing an excellent job at work, but our own health and personal improvement tend to be at the bottom of our to-do lists. That should change from now on. Prioritizing and planning to take time for yourself to work out or to spend more money on coaching is not egotistic or self-centered. Prioritizing your improvement will improve the lives of your loved ones, too.

You must schedule to get things done. Make it a habit to schedule at least forty minutes of uninterrupted "me" time every day. In that time you can exercise, journal, read, relax, or meditate. If you can't find forty consecutive minutes each day for yourself, you can break it in two slots of twenty minutes. So go get your agenda and schedule this time, every day. Make it priority number one.

### 3. Track Your Progress

Bridget Jones, the main character in the book and movie *Bridget Jones's Diary*, weighs herself every day and counts calories the whole day long, and records all of this in her diary to track her progress in her attempt to lose some weight. Did she eat better because of it? On the contrary, she judged herself for eating too many calories, and she sometimes even drank or smoked more to console her feelings of failure.

When we start to count calories and weigh ourselves daily, like Bridget, there is a big chance that we are focusing on the wrong indicators of making progress. If you are used to counting calories all day, I would like to invite you to stop doing that for a while. Of course it makes sense to watch the calories in certain foods. But counting calories is not much fun—nor is being obsessed with a number on the scale! I suggest you use your scale once a week on the same day at the same time.

Use something else to measure your progress. You can use your hands to feel your body getting more toned, the looseness of your clothes as an indicator of weight loss, or the improvement you make in the duration or level of physical exercise.

I have always used matryoshka dolls (Russian nesting dolls) as a way to measure the progress of my weight-loss coaching groups. For every five kilograms my coaching group lost on average, one smaller doll was placed next to the bigger one. This inspired my clients even more than the number on the scale. You could also put beans or other counting objects in a glass every time you work out and treat yourself to a spa treatment when the glass is full. Buy a journal and track your own process that personally motivates you, and you will be able to see the progress that you have made even after one week.

But this book is not just about weight loss; it's about personal growth as well. So how do you measure your progress in personal growth? You will notice an improvement in your relationships, and, most important, you will have a better relationship with yourself. That is a feeling that cannot be measured in pounds but in the amount of time that you are feeling truly happy with who you are, no matter what the circumstances. I aim to feel good about myself twenty-four hours per day, seven days a week.

> ♥ Focus on daily progress, taking the daily action that will lead to results that move you forward. Baby steps on a daily basis can become giant leaps in a few months.
> ♥ Measure your progress in a way that feels best for you. It is not necessary to use the scale daily.

## 4. See This Journey as Practice

If there was a magic pill for permanent weight loss or happiness, a fairy dust powder that would transform us all so that we had a perfect body with perfect character without any challenges, life would be very easy and very, very dull. Let's face it: The problems you have overcome already, the challenges you have faced and conquered, are the moments of life that you cherish. You will always remember the moments you struggled and survived, the moments you wanted to give up but you did not, the moments you stretched yourself to learn and grow. The most precious gifts in life are packed in sandpaper, as motivational speaker Lisa Nichols so beautifully says. And unwrapping those gifts, my dear friend, takes practice.

> See every new task and every new skill you want to learn as practice, and don't judge yourself for failing a few times before you succeed.

Be willing to learn. Remember, the changes you are about to make must be seen as practice, and you will fall off the wagon several times before you succeed. That is normal. The way you react when you do fall off the wagon will determine your success. Mistakes are just lessons to learn, and you should learn in joy. Real failure is the refusal to learn lessons from the mistakes you made in the past—you will probably repeat those until you get the lesson!

Let me ask you: If you saw a five-year-old crying because he fell from his bike, would you judge him for falling and not succeeding at riding a bike the first time? Or would you pick him up, caress him, and whisper that he can try again and that it will all work out fine?

So do you do that for yourself as well? When you fall off the wagon or fail in life, do you nurture yourself and tell yourself that it is okay to fail several times before you succeed? After a weight-loss failure, do you still think you are capable of losing weight? Think back to that five-year-old and compare your reactions to him and to yourself when you fell off your bike in life, when you failed to lose the weight, when you overate when you felt alone. Let go of the guilt and the judgment. Let go of the fear of failure.

When you feel like falling, failing, or forgetting who you are truly meant to be, connect to your nurturing capacities and embrace yourself like you would the five-year-old. Cookies or candy or cake don't care for you. You should learn to care for yourself with your whole heart. You don't have to beat yourself up for not sticking to the suggestions I will make for you. You have to love yourself enough to see failures in life as lessons learned.

In other words, I don't want you to feel deprived; I want you to feel fulfilled. I don't want you to feel scared; I want to you feel confident. I don't want you to feel alone; I want you to always feel good in your own company. Because it matters. It is practice.

## 5. Find the Right People to Support You

A few months ago my daughter, Kiki, and I had an awesome lunch in a tiny Turkish restaurant with our trashmen. (Yes, our trashmen.) They asked if they could join us at the only table on a terrace on a hot summer day. Kiki (who was four years old) was a little bit shy; she had never seen that many tattoos and piercings in her life, nor was she used to their manners, the volume of their voices, and the kind of words they used ("Mummy, what does f*ck actually mean?" she whispered very softly in my ear). She stared at them as if she was seeing water burning. They tried to start a conversation with her, and she flushed. But after they showed her how a big girl should eat a hamburger, she laughed out loud, and the ice was broken.

In that same week I had dinner with a millionaire. The millionaire was dropping famous names and talking and laughing about himself the whole time. I was so much more inspired by our friendly trashmen, who now often wave when they pick up the garbage. The millionaire was fickle and shallow, yet he was supposedly the type of person we should all want to be around. Most people would likely reject the tattooed and pierced trashmen, without refined manners, at first sight, but in truth they were so much more genuine and kind and inspiring.

Always keep your ears and eyes and heart open for new friendships, and don't be afraid to end friendships that are not helping you progress in life but are draining your energy.

Sometimes people can become frightened when you want to change. Please don't let them sabotage your journey. Simply acknowledge them and with love explain the reason behind the change. Stay focused on your own path and goals.

The right people can help you progress so much more, so never be afraid to ask for help. Share your dreams with as many people as possible because you never know who can provide you with the one piece of missing information you need. A lot of people keep their weight-loss attempts private out of fear of failure, but I recommend that you share it as an exciting self-improvement journey instead of a weight-loss attempt.

Surround yourself with uplifting, positive, empowering people. Empower and uplift them too, and happiness and connections will flourish. Create that support team as soon as possible.

> Find the right people to fill the gap inside you to get to your dream, and let them hold you accountable.

# Chapter 4

# TRANSFORM YOUR BODY

Unlike adults, kids can transform themselves within a second. In the Netherlands, children make believe in the past tense: "I was the princess and you were the knight and we had a little baby." The kid who will play the baby is never really, truly satisfied with his role. But he endures the game because on the next turn he might play the knight, king, or dragon.

We all want to transform within a second, and we all want to transform upward. We want to transform ourselves in such way that we feel more important, more loved, more seen. We don't want to shrink backward in the past, but grow upward into our better future, change into the person we know we were meant to be.

Sometimes we even think that our life will finally be great when we have transformed our bodies to a certain size. We will ask for a bigger salary when we fit in a size 10. We will ask for the date when we have lost fifteen pounds. We will feel beautiful when we fit in those jeans. We postpone until X happens, but X never comes. Now is a great time to do what you want and to reveal the best version of you in the meantime. First, I have a little warning for you: Simply reading this chapter will not transform your body. The people who are most successful in changing their lifestyle seek ongoing help in maintenance programs, and they are part of a community of like-minded people.

I want you to have the five most important tools so you can start right away.

## 1. Get Clarity

When you are in a big mall for the first time and you need to find a particular store, you look at the map that shows all the stores and cafés. A big red dot or arrow tells you YOU ARE HERE so you can easily find your way to the store you're seeking.

When you want to transform your body, you have to know your starting point, or your "red dot," before you know which way to turn.

To locate your red dot, you need to know your numbers and your feelings about them. Let me be honest: The total truth about your current physical state is not "served with warm milk and cookies," as Lisa Nichols says. I think the reality might sometimes taste like rotten milk.

That is where your growth begins. Dare to open your eyes fully, see the reality as it is, and how painful it is or how ashamed you might feel about it. Or how much you might have avoided it. The beauty of the red dot is that is gives a clear signal: We will stop being stuck *here,* and start moving toward a new destiny. It's a little flag on the map that says "healthier, happier, and more full of love."

If your red dot could speak it might say, "Overweight; tired; and full of cheap, fast, and easy food." Or it might say, "Not feeling attractive, not expressing inner beauty from the inside out, avoiding mirrors." Or it might say, "Lack of energy; lack of discipline; lack of time, money and will." Whatever your red dot is shouting at you, listen to it carefully, note your numbers, and know that the future will be better. I believe in you. I hope you can see and feel that through my words on these pages.

Before you start losing weight, you also need to get clarity on your intake. Go to turningfatintolove.com to download a diary for you to keep track of everything you eat. During the next week, write down *everything* that goes into your mouth, both liquid and food.

Write down:

- when you eat
- what you eat
- how much you eat
- if you are hungry before you started eating

Before we go further, let us get clear on a few numbers you need to know.

Go to a physician or a physical therapist to have a check-up. Know your numbers and speak with a doctor about your risk factors. He or she should give you proper advice about physical activity and medicine. You must have clarity on what is at stake, and an open conversation with your doctor will help you!

Risk factors to be discussed with a doctor include:

1. Do you smoke?
2. Do you have hypertension?
3. Do you have low HDL cholesterol (serum concentration less than 35 mg/liter)?

4. Do you have an impaired fasting glucose (between 110 and 125 mg/dL)?

5. Do you have a family history of premature coronary heart disease—at or before fifty-five years of age experienced by a first-degree male relative, or sixty-five years of age experienced by a first-degree female relative?

6. Men: Are you older than forty-five?

7. Women: Are you older than fifty-five?

These are the other important numbers to discuss with your doctor:

1. Weight

2. Body mass index (BMI). To calculate BMI using kilograms and meters, divide your weight in meters by the square of your height in kilograms. To calculate your BMI using pounds and inches, divide your weight in pounds by the square of your height in inches, then multiply the result by 703.

3. Waist circumference. A high-risk waist circumference for men is 102 centimeters (40 inches); for women, 88 centimeters (35 inches). A high waist circumference is associated with an increased risk for type 2 diabetes, dyslipidemia, hypertension, and cardiovascular disease in patients with a BMI between 25 and 34.9.

4. Blood pressure

5. Cholesterol (if necessary, let your MD decide)

6. Glucose/ Hba1c (if necessary, let your MD decide)

7. Fat percentage

8. Minutes of daily exercise

9. Hours of sleep

10. How motivated you are on a scale from 1 to 10 to make changes

Make an appointment with your doctor and get clarity. Make a follow-up appointment for two months later. When you have clarity on where you are, it is easier to see where you are going.

## 2. Kitchen Makeover (Before You Get Your Own Makeover)

Not only so you have to go through some changes, your environment does, too. Have you ever seen the home makeovers on *Oprah* done by Nate Berkus? I loved watching those, especially to see what it did for the lucky people involved. Your own makeover starts with a makeover inside the cupboard and fridge.

Throw away anything that is expired or unhealthy (or give the unhealthy food away to someone who wants it). Make a distinctive drawer or cupboard for your partner and children and guests, and fill it with food that they like, not your favorite comfort food. Then fill all your cupboards with healthy food.

Remember: What goes into your shopping cart will disappear in your mouth!

### *Foods That Make You Slimmer, Healthier, and More Beautiful*

Some foods actually help you lose weight more easily when you eat a lot of them. A lot of people are overfed but undernourished. Let us turn that around and give ourselves more of what we really need.

**Eat a lot more vegetables, raw or cooked.** These provide fiber, phytochemicals, and other essential nutrients, and you will be less likely to consume excess calories. The nutrient-packed ones are red, orange, and green. The green leafy vegetables, like Swiss chard, collards, kale, and spinach, are the healthiest, especially when you eat them raw (source for this section: USDA Center for Nutrition Policy and Promotion).

Here are some tips to increase your intake of vegetables:

1.  Add beans and peas more often to salads, main dishes, side dishes, and soups. Beans and peas are great sources of dietary fiber and rich in protein. They can be used as a substitute for meat as well.

2.  Eat a salad for lunch every day. The green leafy vegetables are the most nutrient-dense. You can eat whole wheat bread with it, or a soup. Most of my clients lost the most weight when they started to eat two salads a day with dark leafy vegetables and other raw vegetables, like peppers and red onion. Eat one as a side dish before or during dinner and one as a meal for lunch.

3.  Add colored vegetables to soups, casseroles, and stews. Freeze portions of soups so that you always have healthy options available.

4.  When you make a sandwich, add sliced cucumber, tomato, raw mushrooms, shredded carrots, spinach, or sprouts to it.

5.  When eating out, choose a vegetable as a side dish and request that cooked vegetables be prepared with little or no salt or fat.

6.  Keep raw, cut-up vegetables handy for quick snacks. Use lower-calorie dips such as hummus.

7.  A glass of tomato juice is healthy and delicious.

8.  Steam your vegetables more often.

9.  Mashed cauliflower can be a substitute for mashed potatoes.

**Keep fruit on hand for snacks and meals.** Fruit is delicious fresh or dried. Here are some tips to increase your intake of fruit:

1.  Replace your high-fat and sugary desserts with fresh or frozen fruit like bananas, strawberries, or peaches.

2. Eat fruit as a snack, and make it a habit to have one piece of fruit in your bag with you all the time in case you get hungry.

3. Wash all fruit thoroughly when you get it home so you can always pick a piece right from the bowl.

**Eat more whole grains.** Substitute refined grains in breakfast cereals, bread, pasta, and rice with whole grains. Check the ingredient list for the words "whole" or "whole-grain." Words like "multi-grain," "100 percent wheat," "cracked wheat," or "bran" do not indicate 100 percent whole-grain products, and these products might not even contain any whole grains. Don't be fooled by the color. Look for whole-grain breads, crackers, and pasta and for brown rice. You will be less hungry for a longer time and you will feed your body better.

**Use only low-fat or fat-free dairy products.**

**Drink water or unsweetened, decaffeinated green tea or coffee.** Eliminate all sugary soft drinks. They are not good for your brain or body.

**Reduce your intake of salt.** Stop adding salt to your foods. Season more often with herbs, lime or lemon juice, vinegar, spices, and chiles. Avoid buying prepared meals or frozen pizza; these typically contain a lot of salt.

**Buy lean meat and fish.** Look for chicken or turkey without the skin, and seek out lower-fat cuts of beef and other meats.

If you fill your stomach from now on with these healthier foods, you will lose weight and look beautiful. If you'll be away from your house for the day, take a healthy salad or even soup in a thermos with you.

## 3. The Hunger Game

The hunger game is a game that will teach you to nourish yourself at all levels, both physically and emotionally.

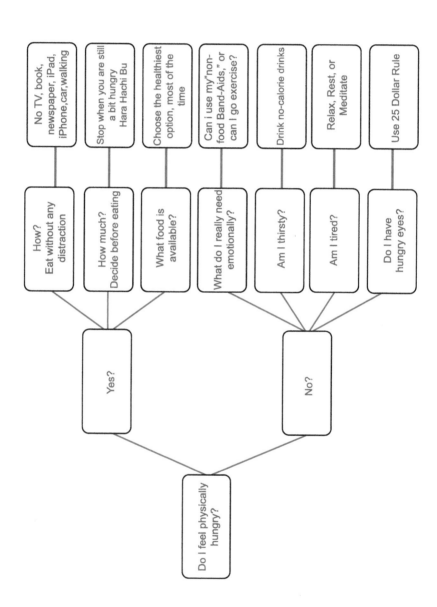

Do I feel physically hungry?

**Yes?**

How?
Eat without any distraction
→ No TV, book, newspaper, iPad, iPhone, car, walking

How much?
Decide before eating
→ Stop when you are still a bit hungry
Hara Hachi Bu

What food is available?
→ Choose the healthiest option, most of the time

**No?**

What do I really need emotionally?
→ Can i use my "non-food Band-Aids," or can I go exercise?

Am I thirsty?
→ Drink no-calorie drinks

Am I tired?
→ Relax, Rest, or Meditate

Do I have hungry eyes?
→ Use 25 Dollar Rule

The goal is to determine whether you are physically hungry or not, what hunger feels like, how much you should eat, how and when you can stop, what to eat, and how to eat, and to learn and notice what you are really hungry for. The outcome is to eat according to your body's needs, to nourish your heart, and to recharge your mind.

This hunger game, by the way, is not a game of winning or losing. This hunger game makes you aware of your options regarding eating and makes you more aware of your body. The more options you have in life, the happier you are. It might be that we all are so used to our own habits that we think that we have only one option available to us given a certain trigger, like when we think we are hungry, we should eat immediately. This is not the case.

Being able to describe the amount of hunger you have and knowing when your body gives the signal "enough" is incredibly difficult for most people. It is like writing in Chinese for Europeans, or understanding Russian for Americans, or reading Braille for seeing people. There is a mismatch, there is a scratch on the CD, so to speak, and we cannot clearly hear the message.

That does not matter. We don't have to recognize our belly hunger before we get rid of the belly fat. We don't have to be able to feel the difference between fatigue and hunger pangs before we start taking care of ourselves. We don't have to recognize that our craving for love is hidden under the craving for chocolate before we start loving ourselves more. We just have to decide to take care of ourselves before we understand every signal that our body gives us.

### Do I Feel Physically Hungry?

*Do I feel physically hungry?* is the first question of the game, before starting to eat. When you have difficulty feeling symptoms of hunger (like most of us do), relax, take a deep breath, and put your hand on your stomach to feel what is going on inside. If you have never felt real hunger because you are always eating to prevent that empty feeling, it might be a good idea to postpone your eating until you feel growling in your belly, just to become aware of the feeling. Normally it takes about three hours after a meal.

Let us first clarify what hunger is *not*.

Hunger can easily be confused with:

- Thirst
- Fatigue
- The reflex of saliva forming in your mouth when thinking of food or seeing food or smelling food
- Pain
- Empty feelings of boredom, loneliness, sadness, unfulfillment, or unattractiveness

Being physically hungry means you can feel the hunger in your body. You are not thinking or desiring or craving, you feel symptoms like those described below.

Hunger calls you when you haven't eaten in about three hours or more.

Hunger calling you might feel like:

- Hunger pangs
- Hollow or empty sensations
- Weakness
- Loss of energy
- Growling
- Trouble concentrating
- Light-headedness
- Headache

- Fatigue
- Irritability

These last three symptoms—headache, fatigue, and irritability—occur and get worse if you postpone eating longer.

If you don't feel hunger symptoms, it is okay.

What is even more important than learning to feel your hunger is this, the most important advice in the whole book when it comes to losing weight: Eat five or six times a day—three healthy meals and three healthy snacks. Eat small amounts of food, and never skip a meal or a snack to make sure you will never get too hungry.

I cannot believe that people who are so used to putting their iPhone on the charger run out of their home to work without breakfast. It is the most important meal of the day, so take time to prepare it and take some time to eat it! I am a big fan of fat-free Greek yogurt, fresh fruit, and some whole-wheat cereals with green tea for breakfast. But feel free to choose your own healthy breakfast using the foods described in the kitchen makeover section above.

Take your time for the next twelve weeks to eat five or six times a day. Notice your hunger feelings. After a while your body will give you hunger signs at the times it is used to getting food. It is more important to eat five or six little portions every day than it is to be able to feel your hunger. But make sure you never get too hungry by skipping meals or snacks, or you will suffer from catch-up hunger all day long.

What is catch-up hunger? Being too hungry will cause you to overeat, and its effects will last longer. You will experience catch-up hunger throughout the whole day! For every meal you skip and every time you don't eat your snacks, you will have the effects coming back to you like an avalanche. You will eat much more than you need when you are too hungry, and you will stay hungry longer than needed. Your DNA was built thousands of years ago, when people needed to hunt and run to prevent starvation, and it has not adapted yet to modern society. Your DNA makes your brain act like you still live in the bush, so when you are too hungry it will think that all the food will be gone soon, that a period of starvation will come, and thus it will create fat reserves quickly for you. But in modern society we generally don't hunt and food is abundant. It is a society in which sometimes the only movement people make all day is using their thumbs for text messaging. Prevent that catch-up hunger by eating regularly, five or six times a day.

Some of you may be thinking, *Yeah, but Pauline, I am allergic to fruits, or I have a special metabolism . . .*

Please! Remove all the "buts" from your vocabulary. They only add fat to your butt. Forgive me being rude.

Back to the hunger game.

### When You Are Physically Hungry

If you answered "yes" to the first question, now ask yourself these three questions: how, how much, and what?

**1. How do I eat?** We are all multitaskers, and we all try to do many things at the same time. Eating while reading. Talking while listening. Eating while driving. Picking up the ringing phone while making love. (Let it ring!) Eating while watching the news. And do you know how many mobile phones are destroyed because they fall into the toilet? What is the reason for taking your mobile phone there? (Maybe you are scared to be alone, or you want to call 911 in case you discover a lost crocodile in your toilet?)

And in the evening, after all this multitasking and working, we sit on the couch in front of the television, zoning out. Sitting tired on the couch, we forget that we still can generate energy from within, we forget who we were meant to be, who we are becoming. We might feel numb because we don't have any energy left. We forget how to plug into our own power, so we plug in to the power of the TV, the iPad, the candy, and the chips, and we eat, we watch, but we are mindless. And that is good, once in a while.

It makes perfect sense. However, if you are still committed to becoming yourself at your highest level, if you are still committed to changing your life and the lives of your loved ones by setting a terrific example, sitting on the couch and eating is a loud signal for change.

From now on, when you are eating, stop all distractions. It is impossible to taste the food properly when you are playing a video game or watching TV. Your body will scream at you that it has had enough, but you will be deaf to its cries while watching the news. When you overeat, your body has no choice but to turn that excess of food directly into fat. Turn that fat into love again by taking care of yourself, by paying attention to your food and your true needs. Eat mindfully in the moment, taste the food instead of the words of the TV host, pay attention to *your* body instead of the people's bodies on your screen. Make your meals a little party—you are worth that. When you feel that sitting and eating mindlessly after dinner is the only option left, be compassionate with yourself and ask yourself what it would take for you to change this. How can this be better? Maybe call a friend, take a walk, take a shower and go to sleep early, meditate, write, clean a drawer, paint . . .

Mothers, especially working mothers, especially single working mothers, who manage their lives and those of their children, have to expend a giant amount of energy to do so, but they can be so depleted at the end of the day that they just give in, give up, and intentionally forget that they are still able to take excellent care of themselves 24/7 in order to recharge their battery. Working men, working women, fathers, grandfathers, and grandmothers can all feel this, too.

In my life, it happened only when the kids were sleeping, after my divorce. The business of giving them a bath, putting them in their pajamas, brushing their teeth, and reading them a great story was such a contrast to the silence that followed afterward. I really enjoyed being able to relax after a busy day of working, cooking, cleaning, and caring, but I felt empty, too, sitting on the couch by myself in silence. So I began to eat candy. On the couch. Watching TV. Without thinking. Soon I realized that for the first time, I had done what I had taught so many people not to do. *I had devoured a whole can of candy without tasting one bite.*

Mindless eating makes us unaware of portion sizes, unaware of taste, temperature, texture, and smell. Young kids never eat mindlessly; they are very present in the moment when they eat.

If you have children, always make sure that eating dinner is a safe and happy family moment for them, not full of stress or distraction. Relax! Let them tell their stories of the day, and share your experiences. Never, ever force a child to eat for fear of punishment or by rewarding with dessert. Make it fun. Say that the broccoli wants to play hide-and-seek in your child's tummy, or that the beans are little sausages. Make a face with the food on the plate, or play a game of who can eat the most beans in the next minute. Let them eat with their hands; when children are young, eating healthily is more important than eating tidily. It is so important for kids to learn to love healthy food instead of being forced to eat it. A child will never starve himself, so have faith and be intelligent in what you offer before dinner. Sometimes it is smart to start with vegetables when he is really hungry, or to offer applesauce next to them for the first twelve times they eat a new vegetable they don't like.

To summarize:

♥ Eat without distractions—that includes iPhones, iPads, TV, newspapers, books, and driving a car.

♥ Make an effort to set the table nicely, especially when you are alone.

♥ Be very compassionate with yourself when you find yourself eating mindlessly. Ask yourself how you can make that situation better, so it will not happen again. Take action on that answer!

**2. How much?** In Okinawa, Japan, a lot of people are more than hundred years old, while the younger generation suffers from obesity. A lot of research has been done to discover why. The younger generation adopted a Western lifestyle, and the older generation stuck to their old eating habits. We can learn a lot from this!

These healthy and happy centenarians eat a plant-based, nutrient-dense diet rich in colors with a lot of tofu and fish. But it is not only what they eat. The real secret to their longevity is found in what they don't eat. They take a moment before dinner and say, *"Hara hachi bu,"* and they clap. It is a Confucian-inspired adage and it means eat until you are 80 percent full. It is staggeringly successful in helping you lose weight. The trick is to decide consciously when to stop eating before you have even started.

The fullness signal that our body gives us is delayed by fifteen to twenty minutes, so we know that when we stop eating, our feeling of satisfaction or fullness will increase in a little while. Most of us overeat because we don't like to wait a little while. We prefer to eat until we have cleaned the plate, until the bag is empty, until there is no ice cream left in the box, until we feel so full that we need to loosen up our trousers, adjust our belt, roll from our chair, and long for a nap on the couch in front of the TV. And when we lie there, we need something with sugar, too. Preferably chocolate, please. Or candy.

When our body is working like crazy to digest all those things it did not ask for, we will get tired and we will crave even more sugar. This occurs when glucose is absorbed very quickly and the body reacts by releasing excessive amounts of insulin to lower the glucose levels. Chances are high that when you experience an after-dinner dip, you did not eat a side salad or whole wheat pasta or brown rice. If you want to prevent an after-dinner dip, eat more healthily and eat less, never until you are overfull. You might want to use visual signs as a signal; for example, when you have eaten half of your plate, check in with your stomach again to feel your state.

*Hara hachi bu* in real life means to stop eating when you are still a bit hungry, when you still would like to eat a few more bites. You don't have to clean the plate. It can feel like a waste to throw food away in the garbage bin, but to use your body as a garbage bin is worse! From now on, remind yourself that you are not a trash can. When you feel like overeating, remind yourself of those healthy, happy hundred-year-old people in Okinawa, who show us that eating less and healthier is worth a lifetime of happiness and vitality.

When you are a little hungry, you need to eat just a little. Sometimes even a few bites are enough to satisfy your belly.

As part of this question, you also need to ask yourself, *How do I stop eating?* Knowing how to stop eating is almost as important as knowing when to start, so here are some suggestions for you.

- Put your napkin over your plate. (Hiding works; just don't start to play hide and seek.)
- Put the plate under water in the sink.
- Walk outside for fifteen minutes.
- Sometimes it helps to clean the kitchen before taking a second helping. It gives you just enough time to feel fully satisfied.

**3. What am I going to eat?** What you choose to eat depends on what is available to you and what you need.

You are 100 percent responsible for what food is available to you, and I would encourage you to fill your environment with healthy food as described earlier. Learn to prepare your meals and snacks ahead of time when you know you won't have a chance to eat healthily at the place where you are going. Everything you put in your mouth will affect your body, heart, and mind.

Choose foods that will help you move forward through the life of your dreams. Don't choose foods that will end up creating a nightmare. You are worthy of living a vital, healthy life. Why would you allow yourself to eat in a way that shows you don't care about yourself, or that you don't care enough about others who would profit from your change? Don't count calories, but love yourself and others so much that you finally decide that you deserve the healthiest and freshest food and drinks, most of the time. You deserve your best body.

Make it a habit to choose one level healthier than you feel like. Your kids (if you have them) will profit their entire lifetime from this; they will see a living example of someone choosing healthy over easy, and it will be tattooed on their brains forever, so that even their kids will profit from you making this choice. Your choices now can be a legacy forever. Just choose the healthiest option most of the time.

What is the healthiest option? Foods that are living are always healthier than refined products. Fruit, vegetables, whole-wheat grains and cereals, and fat-free dairy are your number-one choices. Second are fruit juices or dried fruits; vegetables with added fat and sauces; white refined bread, rice, and pasta; taco shells; pancakes; and waffles. Third are ice-milk bars, frozen fruit juice bars, low-fat frozen yogurt, and baked chips.

The last choice—and you will have to want to pay twenty-five dollars for these—are cookies, cakes, pies, ice cream, chocolate, candy, chips, buttered microwave popcorn, fried potatoes, croissants, muffins, doughnuts, sweet rolls, hot dogs, fried chicken, and the like. You still can eat them, but only once in a while, and in small portions. And if you eat them, *enjoy them and eat slowly!*

*When You Are Not Physically Hungry*

When you are not physically hungry but you still feel like eating, ask yourself these four questions:

**1. What do I need emotionally?** Try to give it to yourself, or go exercise! When you feel mad, sad, bored, deprived, unloved, unworthy, or guilty, food can be your best friend. It does not judge you, it does not yell at you, it does not leave you, and it always tastes delicious. Since you were a baby, food was nourishment but also love and care. The problem with this friend is that it will leave you alone in the end, feeling even more sad, deprived, unworthy, or guilty. It is a false, fast friend, not healthy for your soul and body. It is a disposable friend, a mirage. So dare to see this truth and dare to ask yourself honestly if eating food has helped you in any way to fix your emotional problems.

You are becoming yourself in your best version, and this coping mechanism is not serving you. So reread chapter 1 and supersize your heart. Then learn to give to yourself what you need the most from others. It is easier said than done, and you might as well consider some counseling to help you get rid of old patterns and problems.

Further, make a food-free area in the house where you have objects or hobbies directly accessible that you love, so that when you have the desire to eat emotionally you have other options immediately available. One of my clients loved to paint, so she rearranged one room in her house in such a way that she could go paint immediately when she felt like eating emotionally. It helped her tremendously, and her urge to binge disappeared.

Another client always carried a bottle of water, a magazine, and nail polish in her bag so that when she felt bored and wanted to eat, she had other options available to her. You could write, or make a call, or do whatever appeals to you that will keep you from heading for the kitchen.

> ♥ Name five things you can do to create a food-free alternative that you love and that is accessible in your house immediately. These are your food-free bandages. Create a few to carry in your bag, too. Be creative.
>
> ♥ What did you love to do when you were young? Is it something you can do again now? I loved biking as a child, and now, when I don't feel good, I will jump on my bike for forty minutes. I feel so much better afterward.

Never underestimate the power of exercise when you have an off day, an off week, or just an off hour. It might be the last thing on earth you want to do; you might much rather give in and indulge yourself in chocolate and candy. But don't forget that you have a Pause button on your forehead! You are capable of postponing your first impulse and using your Pause button to stop you from acting mindlessly. The fact that you are not used to pushing Pause does not mean you should ignore the button now. If your food-free bandages don't work, if you are about to open the bag, push the button and remind yourself of your dreams and of who you need to become to get there. Then just walk away; change your environment. If it is possible, walk outside, and keep on walking and walking for a while, as if you left the house to get some milk but never returned. But do come back! Come back refreshed, replenished, positive, and optimistic. The urge to eat will have disappeared into the fresh air outside. If you really have a winner's mentality, go do a fitness class or video and sweat it all out. Your craving for sugar and fat will disappear, and you will not only look better but also feel better.

**2. Am I thirsty?** Hunger can also easily be confused with thirst. When you are really thirsty, your body has been dehydrated for a while and the signal is delayed. Thirst should be prevented. Drink small bottles of water or drink (green) tea without sugar, all day long. Your skin will profit too: you will look beautiful and younger.

**3. Am I tired?** When we are tired, we often eat way too much sugar, because glucose is the only fuel for the brain. We want to fuel the engine, and it feels like a hunger that cannot be postponed or satisfied with something like yogurt or fish or raw vegetables. On the contrary, we want cookies and candy, and a lot of them. The remedy to this is to rest instead of drinking more caffeine or eating sugar. Because your body did not ask for it (but your tired mind did), your body won't give a signal that it has had enough! So sleep more or meditate or take it easy; it can make a difference of fourteen pounds of fat a year.[4] Don't look for things outside to fix problems inside. You can not expect sugar or other people to refuel your tank! You are responsible for resting enough so your battery will recharge.

**4. Am I looking with hungry eyes?**

If you are not hungry but you have hungry eyes, because you see the most delicious food in front of you, be careful. Don't eat it anyway; only eat it if you are willing to pay twenty-five dollars for it. Only eat it if it is the best of the best.

I don't like designating forbidden foods, because everything that is forbidden rises immediately to number one on your desire list. It is like me saying to a child, "Please do not look in that black velvet box over there, because it is private," and then expect her not to look. If I had not mentioned it, she likely would never have noticed it. It is human nature to desire the unavailable.

So, there is no forbidden chocolate or chips or cake. However, you have to raise the standard for your taste. You can eat the chocolate only if it is the best of the best: if it is from a world-class shop or

---

4    "Dr. Oz's 4-Step Weight Loss Plan You Can Do in Your Sleep," Oprah.com, http://www.oprah.com/health/How-to-Lose-Weight-While-You-Sleep-Dr-Oz, accessed May 5, 2013.

brand, if it is flown in from Switzerland, or if it is handmade in a restaurant. You are becoming you at a world-class level. So, if you indulge, indulge only in food at a world-class level. You should be willing to pay twenty-five dollars for it. And then enjoy it! With gusto, with all your senses, taste it, smell it, feel the texture in your mouth, and enjoy the tasting experience, *slowly.* When you actually taste your food, you won't need as much of it to feel satisfied. Don't do this too often, of course. Once a week, or once every two weeks. Taste small portions at a low frequency and savor it.

Otherwise, it is a waste of money, a waste of your taste, and even a waste of your life. If you keep choosing easy over healthy, you are wasting years of your life, and the lives of your loved ones who will need to take care of you when you become ill. I know I sound harsh, but it is the inconvenient truth that will set you free, finally.

All other low-class junk food—resist it until a better time. A better time is when your health is so vibrant and so in balance that there is more space for unhealthy food. Not now, though.

Get used to playing the hunger game and remember that you don't have to be able to feel all your different kinds of hunger or satisfaction immediately before starting to nourish yourself properly. Expand your options every time you feel like eating and make it a habit to choose the best one most of the time. (I repeat: most of the time.) Expanding and becoming aware of the different options you have in every moment will help you make a better choice in any situation.

## 4. Exercise

*Those who think they have not time for bodily exercise*
*will sooner or later have to find time for illness.*

—Edward Stanley

Sometimes we all feel restless. We want to move, to fly; we feel the need to fill our lungs with fresh air, stretch our muscles, and maybe even do a secret dance in the streets. But sometimes our body forces us to slow down, to find balance, or to rest because it is too tired or maybe ill.

Or, more likely, our mind tells us that it is not convenient to move our body more, that we should be ashamed of our body in a swimsuit, that we don't have enough time or money, that the weather is not good enough, that the astrology signs are not right, that the moon is in the wrong position. So we make a promise to ourselves: tomorrow we will start. Really. Tomorrow will be the day. But tomorrow never comes; tomorrow stays tomorrow forever. Tomorrow stays tomorrow, and tomorrow never dies.

Having MS has forced me to live life often with the handbrake on, to walk more slowly instead of running fast, to take a healthy nap instead of going out and dancing.

But I danced with my fears, I ran from other-love to self-love, and finally—finally—was able to fly to my dreams. In doing so I had to exercise my body. Being the overweight director of a successful weight management institute did not help my credibility. Being overweight did not help me feeling good enough to help other overweight people.

When I first supersized my heart, I did not need food to feel better anymore, because I felt better from within. Then I began to focus on my thinking and no longer allowed my thoughts to sabotage me. And finally, I made a plan.

My plan was to learn to run in fifteen weeks, three times a week. It started with two minutes of running alternated with one minute of walking. It ended with twenty-five minutes of running and three minutes of walking. In the end I mastered the miles effortlessly. I was running from my village to the one nearby.

I have been told that I have changed the lives of my clients or inspired my friends to be better people. I am very proud of that. Starting my own business when the doctors said I was too ill to work made me proud. Graduating from Wageningen University and getting the title "engineer" made me proud, because it was challenging for me, not being good at math. When Kiki says she loves me more than all the animals, grasses, butterflies, and stars in the world, and Daan gives me a thousand kisses mixed with snot, I feel extremely proud and loved.

But one of the personal things that I am most proud of is the gap I bridged between my current reality and my dream future. That gap became closer, the longer I could run from my home to another village nearby. The more fit I was, the better I could activate my dreams.

I remember running and thinking, *I am doing it! I am following my dreams! I am moving forward with my life, creating a healthier future.* I felt free, I felt proud, and I looked beautiful.

And I had to go deep, very deep, to be able to do so. I get out of bed at six o'clock, do my Pilates in front of the TV, drink water, take a bottle with me, and I run through life like Forrest Gump.

Still, every morning that the alarm clock rings, I do not want to get out of my warm bed. I have to accept all the uncomfortable feelings that come with creating new habits, like strong resistance, or fear of failure or change, and bust boldly through them. It sometimes feels like being stuck in traffic, wanting to push the Fast Forward button, but in the beginning the Pause button was the only option.

Step by step, minute by minute, I grew stronger, and not just in my legs and in my heart. My mind began to believe that I was able to do anything, everything. That is a gift you can give yourself, too. You don't have to run to another village to feel proud of yourself and believe in yourself. But you have to do something that you thought you could not do and simply take the first step. Maybe you want a personal trainer but don't feel comfortable hiring one. Or maybe you want to get slimmer and your doctor advises that exercising in water is best for you, but you don't like swimming because you feel embarrassed to put on a swimsuit. Just try it eleven times, and see if you feel better. In the things we resist the most are often hidden opportunities for growth.

Make exercise part of your daily ritual, and make it part of your life. Please do it, because your better future depends on it.

> ♥ Go to a physical therapist to get good advice on what is best for your body.
> ♥ Find a friend who is more active than you who can join you.
> ♥ Set the alarm clock on your phone for the three times you get up early to exercise each week for a few weeks into the future. Decide that nothing can stop you.
> ♥ Make it easy for yourself to move more by putting the treadmill in the living room instead of letting it gather dust in the attic. Put it in front of the TV; there must be one or two shows or the news that you watch daily. Use that time to burn calories.
> ♥ Have your exercise clothes near you, your fitness shoes in your car, and an umbrella, your iPod, and some water with you at all times, so that when you are on the road you still can find time to exercise or walk. Or make sure you have a jump rope when you are on the road; jumping for even five minutes will increase your metabolism. Be prepared!

When you implement exercise as a daily routine, you will notice that you will not only feel and look better, but also sleep better!

## 5. Sleep like a Baby

When you start to exercise more, you will sleep better. We all need a minimum of seven to eight hours of sleep. Too little sleep can have adverse effects on your health without you realizing it. When you sleep less than you need, you gain fat, you weaken your immune system, and your memory will be impaired.

Here are some tips for sleeping better:

1.  Make it a habit to sleep in complete darkness, because your brain will interpret light as a signal for action. You have your own circadian rhythm, and your internal clock will be disrupted if you have light in your bedroom.
2.  Leave your window open, no matter how cold it is. Fresh air makes you sleep and breathe better.
3.  Use earplugs in your ears when your environment is too noisy.
4.  The optimal room temperature for sleep is between sixty and sixty-eight degrees Fahrenheit. Your body drops in temperature four hours after sleeping, so some scientists believe that mimicking this improves your sleep.
5.  Reserve your bed for sleeping, not working or watching TV. It is harder to relax in bed when you are accustomed to working in it.
6.  Set your alarm clock at night seven to eight hours before you need to wake up, if you have problems going to bed on time— as opposed to using the alarm clock to get up on time!
7.  Wear warm socks; cold feet might cause you to wake up at night.
8.  Journal or read or meditate before sleeping, or do a combination of those.
9.  Avoid coffee and heavy meals or snacks before going to bed. Your last snack before sleep should be consumed several hours before bedtime.

10. Take a bath or shower as part of your bedtime ritual.
11. Listen to relaxation CDs.

When you give yourself this healthy and precious package of sleeping well, eating healthily, and exercising consistently, you will thrive. But the bonus will work as a catalyst. That bonus is body love.

## Body Love as a Bonus

Love is not about perfection but about acceptance. Loving your body is courageous, by the way; almost nobody does it properly (including myself).

No cream, no massage, and no diet can do for your body what you can do when you start to love yourself and your body, just the way it is now, even before improvements. You will better take care of yourself.

Spoil your body by giving it only healthy food for the next three months. Cheat only on occasions that you plan on your calendar.

Spoil your body by starting to exercise daily.

And welcome Mr. Discomfort any time, any place. He will be your guest on your journey. Welcome and embrace him, because he will help you turn fat into love. The struggle of having him around you is nothing compared to the struggle you have put your body through over the years. Mr. Discomfort has a very ugly face, a disgusting odor, and rude behavior. It does not feel comfortable to be around this guy; hence his name. It feels like giving up, giving in, and running away. Welcome these feelings, and then release them.

So when you are procrastinating on exercising, when you want to choose easy over healthy, when you forget to stop when you have had enough, know that that is Mr. Discomfort talking to you. Welcome him, expect him, and *push through*. He is also very tricky in letting you believe the lie that your body should be more perfect.

Learn how to take perfect care of your body instead of judging your body for not being perfect. Your body is a classroom, not a courtroom. It is about adoring and appreciating and pouring love in, not about throwing garbage in it or treating it like trash. Your body is a temple, not a trash can. Your body is your home for the rest of your life.

Loving your body is not about perfection but about acceptance and care. I understand your fears, your doubts, and your misconceptions, but beauty does not come in one size or one shape. I know you want to lose excess fat, but you will lose that weight more easily when you start to accept your body as it is now.

Here are some numbers about your body, so you can appreciate it more:

- We have more connections in our brains than stars in the universe.
- Per second the body produces 25 million new cells—that is, the entire population of Canada—per second!
- Every five months your body renews your liver.
- Every month your skin is renewed.
- Every two weeks the mucus layer of the stomach renews itself.

Your body is working really hard for you to live your life fully. Where you put your attention is what grows. Vice versa for your body: It will try to get your attention by growing and growing. It craves your good care. It has a hunger for health and energy. It is thirsty for water instead of soft drinks or fruit juices.

Your body does not want to be lazy, but it was forced by you to sit on the couch, and you could no longer fit into your clothes. Your body was made to carry you, not to cage you. It never wanted that. Never. But you stopped listening to its voice.

When you became deaf to its true needs, it had no other choice than to turn your absence of love into fat so that you would listen again. And love again. And care again.

And it is more difficult now than ever, because your body has changed. It is not the way it was before you forgot to take care of it. But it is not too late to step up.

Show some body love today. Yes, you should eat more healthily. Yes, you should exercise a whole lot more. But don't forget healing touch. Your body deserves that, possibly after a while of neglect and judgment. So get a massage or a scrub, or buy a fancy body lotion so you can feel you have a body from the neck down, not only from the neck up.

When you start to appreciate and take care of your body, it will reward you after some time. It will reveal itself in the most energetic and vital way possible. It will be thankful that you acknowledge its existence, that you listen to its needs, and that you take action to help it function, instead of sabotaging it in every way. And you know what? When you start to take excellent care of your body, you will inspire others to do the same.

# Chapter 5

# CHANGE THE WORLD
# BUT BEGIN WITHIN

Have you ever noticed that when someone you know changes successfully, you become more inspired to do the same? Have you ever noticed that when one family member starts to improve their eating habits, suddenly the whole family benefits from that change and starts to live in more healthy ways? Have you ever noticed that when *you* change, it inspires others?

You can help others make progress. You can give others hope by being a great example, and they might think: "If he or she can do it, I believe that I can do it, too."

Strive to become that role model, even if you still have to begin your own journey. Encourage others to live more healthy lives, just by living out your new habits and sharing your results. Inspire others to live a life full of love, just by expressing an abundance of love for them, for yourself, and for your life. It makes you a rock star. It makes you popular. It makes you feel successful.

Become an inspiring role model for your loved ones in your life, just by changing yourself. Step up so that they can follow.

I have had my own role models in my life, and one that had the most impact was my grandfather, whom I mentioned earlier in chapter 1.

In this last chapter I will tell his story, and I hope it will inspire you to think about the kind of story you are writing right now with your life and your behavior.

An old Roman saying goes: "Every family should have one elder to take care of, and when you don't have one you should buy one."

My grandfather, Dr. Wilhelm Marten Westerman, was a highly respected surgeon and anesthetist in Haarlem. Grandfather lost his wife to cancer when they had been married for thirty years. After living alone for years, he remarried when he was seventy-nine. But at age eighty-five he divorced, because his new wife was much more interested in his money than his love, and even though he was at this advanced age, he did not want to spend the last years of his life with her, knowing that she did not really love him. After his divorce, he came to live with my parents, my older sister, and me.

Every day around 5 p.m., I would walk to the attic with a little piece of cheese in one hand and a glass of port in the other. Grandfather would sit at his desk, reading or taking notes, as I would knock three times and then silently open the door. He was always glad to see me. He kissed me and immediately moved to another chair with help of his cane. I would put the cheese and port next to him at the table, and then take off the warm bedcover and spread it over his knees. Then I would sit down on the floor and enjoy our time together, listening, learning, and laughing together.

I loved those afternoons, when he would tell me everything about how the heart and the blood worked, about history, or about books. He told his stories with an incredible sense of humor and intelligence. I learned so much from his teachings.

More importantly, he taught me by example that you are never, ever too old to change your life completely and become the happiest person you have ever been.

With a magnifying glass he read the newspaper, and every day he made notes. When he was eighty-six, he still biked through the village, and many of our family and friends knew exactly the route he used to bike. Sometimes, when it started to rain, we would have to go out to look for him (at that time there were no mobile phones), and most of the time he had found a shelter under a tree or in a tunnel, or he was invited into a warm house for coffee by a friend of my mother's. When we came to pick him up he had a big smile on his face, and he waved proudly for having survived nature again. He loved his life, he loved people, and he took excellent care of himself. He ate very healthily, he exercised, and he washed his hands like only a surgeon does. Until he died at the age of ninety-three, he was an inspiring man who lived and loved life to the fullest.

If you can listen to your heart at the age of eighty-five, decide to divorce, and start all over again—if you have enough self-love to take excellent care of yourself and dedicate your life to learning and sharing your wisdom and love—then you have succeeded in life and have become an inspiring and happy role model. My grandfather's example proves that change is possible at all ages, at all sizes, and at any time. But if you are not eighty-five yet, please don't wait until you are to take excellent care of yourself, because that might be too late.

When you are near the end of your life, sitting in your rocking chair with a little child in front of you, what story about your life do you want to tell? And what example are imprinting on that little child through your behavior? Today you can start to write the story you want to tell that child by beginning to *live it now*. By breathing it. By deciding to do it.

You have everything within you—everything it takes to be the most happy and healthy version of you. Begin within. Start without diets or shakes. Love and accept yourself first. You have so much love and energy within, more than you can spend in three lifetimes. Begin within. You have the highest and best version of yourself within, waiting to be unpacked, waiting to be revealed, waiting to see the light of the world. Begin within. You don't have to change yourself; you just have to accept yourself and all your miracles within. You are not broken; you don't need to be fixed. Begin within. You don't need to lose weight before you can love yourself; you need to love yourself and therefore take excellent care of yourself. Nothing less than the highest standard for your loved ones, nothing less than the highest standard for you. When you cannot accept a part of you, you will always sabotage your own joy, your own progress, your own success.

You can make the amazing decision today to make a difference in so many other lives by living a life that is full of energy and love for yourself. You can make a contribution to others just by being a terrific example and a great source of support.

None of us can guarantee that we'll be here tomorrow, no matter what age we are. Commit to making a change, however small, *today*.

Your remarkable decision to transform your body, to supersize your heart, and to grow your brain can have an effect on others that you have no idea of now.

Be the change. It will have a giant ripple effect, like throwing a pebble in a pond.

Whether you want to help other people to change themselves or you want to help yourself, always come from a place of compassion and love. Forget about judgments, forget about punishment. Look with compassionate eyes, listen with compassionate ears, and help with an abundance of dedication to let the other person (and yourself) succeed in their transformation.

*We can't help being thirsty, moving toward the voice of the water.*
—Jalal ad-Din Rum, Persian poet (1207–1273)

To illustrate the importance of self-care and self-love, here is another story:

A young man was lost in the desert, and he was so thirsty that he thought he would go insane. Then a generous older man offered him a half mug of water. The younger man was so happy that he jumped up to embrace the old man. But the old man felt weak himself, and the glass fell out of his shaky hands and the water was gone.

The message behind it is this: First provide more than enough for yourself, so you can serve others from the overflow.

We are all thirsty sometimes, and not only for water. We want more energy, we want more happiness, and we want more love.

The older man was certainly generous, but he was only able to give a half mug of water out of his resources. If you were in the desert a whole day and were very thirsty, and you were offered a half glass of water, you would take it, wouldn't you? But your thirst would not be quenched by half a glass of water. The thirst would expand rapidly in your body. After a little while you would begin to feel weak, fatigued, and worried, and you might even have a headache, with a very dry tongue and mouth.

Now imagine that someone led you to a waterfall, with fresh drinkable water. You feel like you could drink the entire waterfall, you are so thirsty. An abundance of fresh, cold water is flowing over you. It never stops, even when you have drunk more than enough; there is enough left. You feel fresh, replenished, and energetic again.

We all need waterfalls to recharge, but somehow it seems so difficult to find them in the "desert" of our busy lives. We have our half glasses, but we need more, and we look around us, thirsty and needy. So why don't we try to create a waterfall ourselves instead of looking outside for more energy, more health, and more love? If we need to recharge ourselves immediately, the waterfall should never be too far away. In fact, it should flow through us so we can provide for others from the overflow and still have more than enough for ourselves.

How do you create or, even better, become an energetic fresh waterfall, when you feel like a stuck, dry river? I hope this book gave you the answer to that question. From a place of self-care and self-love, make your health a priority in your life, and this approach will transform you from the inside out.

For your convenience, here is a summary of how to supersize your heart, grow your brain, and transform your body.

Supersize your heart with these seven ingredients:

1. Self-love. When you accept yourself and your body completely, it is easier to change. Otherwise, borrow the loving, compassionate eyes of others to see your own beauty more clearly and accept their love unconditionally. No matter what your size or accomplishments, you are enough.
2. Authenticity. When you are who you truly are, not who others want you to be, you will be so much happier. Show your brightest and your darkest sides—it is okay, because it is you.
3. High-quality connections. The people around you can lift you up or they can drain your energy or even sabotage your dreams.

Make it a point to develop high-quality friendships by being the best friend possible, and don't invest too much in friends that don't help you succeed.

4. Passion. Ignite the passion in your life again by doing more of what you love to do. Engage fully in each moment and be and act enthusiastic.

5. Gratitude. Be thankful and grateful every day and express your gratitude for others. Think of three things you are grateful for every day before sleeping.

6. Let go of the past. Live in the present moment and forgive those who are holding you hostage—not to help them, but to help yourself. Let go and start your exciting life.

7. Positivity and inspiration. Inspire yourself, inhale love, and exhale positivity, and you will attract so many wonderful people that your heart will grow.

Self-love is the most important of these. If you don't feel good enough about yourself, life is more difficult. You don't need to change or lose weight to love or to feel loved. You don't have to be in a relationship to love or to feel loved. You may lose your partner, you may have gained weight, but you never lose your love and your power. Please, dispel this spell you are under, this illusion of not being good enough, of not being thin enough to accept love effortlessly and unconditionally. Please wake up from this scary hypnosis of expecting rejection or needing the approval of others. Wake up now to the truth: that you are worthy, that you are loved, that you are enough now and forever.

You can connect to your power inside, and you can connect to your heart power as well. Your heart is supersized now, and it will help you recognize your own lovability, the beauty of your body, and the beauty and the importance of your voice.

I have struggled with all of the above, especially accepting that my voice mattered, that I had beauty within that should shine through, and that I don't need love from others to love myself. Please don't let my struggle become yours. Show up in the world with no restrictions and care for yourself enough so that your future self will be thankful you did. Never let your thoughts and actions cost you your health, vitality, or self-esteem. Self-care and self-love will save the lives of others. Live it, breathe it, teach it, and sweat it.

Grow your brain with these five steps:

1. Take 100 percent responsibility. Own your fat. No matter what, you are responsible for your life, body, and health. Knowing this gives you tremendous power and freedom. No diet, shake, or guru can change your body or your happiness about life. Only you can.

2. Talk about what you want instead of what you don't want. Don't talk fat. It is really important for success that you dream the dream and talk about it, most of the time. Don't focus on things that are not going well. Focus your energy and time on what you want to achieve.

3. Take action. Every day, do something that will help you get forward. Track your progress.

4. Let go of unconscious fear. Turn on the light. If you feel that you are sabotaging yourself in getting what you want, it might be that your unconscious mind is blocking you. Find resources to help you—like Holosync meditation, for example.

5. Implement the seven-step Big Brain Plan. Really work this plan, not only for your brain but also for the beauty of your skin.

Transform your body with the following five steps:

1. Know exactly where you are right now. Have a candid conversation with your doctor about your numbers and track your intake of both fluids and food.
2. Give your kitchen a makeover. Make sure that you have healthy food available not only in your kitchen but everywhere you go. Make it a habit to prepare healthy meals to take with you when you are on the road and may not be sure if you can choose healthy options. Think of salads and soups and fresh vegetables and fruit more often.
3. Play the hunger game. Read this section a few times to know how, how much, what, and when to eat: little portions of healthy food five or six times a day. Make sure you have your food-free bandages and a food-free zone in your house for when you feel like eating but are not hungry. Also, be aware of all the things hunger can be confused with, like tiredness or thirst or just the thought of food.
4. Exercise. It is the best antidepressant ever: it will make you lose weight faster, and you will look so much better when you commit to daily exercise. Try walking, biking, swimming, yoga, or Pilates. Choose something that you like, and get support if necessary. Overcome your excuses. You are turning fat into love. You are changing yourself and your world.
5. Sleep enough. Enough sleep is so important and so overlooked as an important tool in weight loss. Not only will your body benefit, but your brain and skin will, too. Relaxation and meditation are helpful. Read chapter 4 again for tips.
6. Bonus: Body love. Spoil your body more often from now on, with massages, body lotions, scrubs, and so on. Your body is not a courtroom; stop judging it and start caring for it.

To transform your body you have to take action on a daily basis. This might cause a lot of discomfort in the beginning and sometimes even arouse negative emotions. Be uncomfortable, be scared, be angry, be doubtful—but do it, no matter what. You should expect Mr. Discomfort. He will transform into Mr. Habit, after a while, but he will still show up as Mr. Discomfort from time to time. Expect that and accept that. Expecting and accepting discomfort is your sacrifice to become the most lovable, most energetic, and most beautiful version of you. When you are going to lose weight, when you are changing your actions, thoughts, and even feelings, it will be messy for a while. The reward is worth it!

Connect with your power again by creating energy in your body, not by trying to find it outside in coffee or Coca-Cola. This power is the part of you that takes action, that will get things done, that is determined to get you energetic again. Let this part of you become more dominant in your life. This inward power will increase your life, strength, and outward power if you have the guts to connect with it again and to stop your self-pity, stop your excuses, and start living more vibrantly and energetically. Dare to strive for more energy, and you will receive so much more as a result.

Being overweight not only changes how we feel about ourselves, but also impacts our health in such a way that it has impact on the lives of others.

Your sacrifice now will not only reward your body later, but also be imprinted in the minds of others around you. Just as my father predicted my best future on that day that I lost hope, I'm going to predict your future even without knowing you: If you work this book instead of just reading it, your future will be full of love and energy. Anything is possible. Even when it seems impossible.

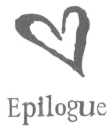

# Epilogue

# SAFE TRAVELS

In this world, in this day and age, more people are dying from the results of obesity and overweight than of hunger. It is overwhelming. It should be changed. All deaths related to bad lifestyle habits should be prevented. I know—I have big dreams.

If you are reading this page, you are probably inspired to change. I am here to remind you of who you are, I am here to remind you of who you need to become (that is *you* to your highest potential), and I am here to say to you that I believe in you. I believe in your strength, in your courage, in your love. I stand next to you when I see your fears, your doubts, your feelings of deprivation. Your past does not equal your future. I am proud of you when I already see who will emerge—the authentic you, with more energy. Be the change. Do not let others steal your health, and please do not become a thief of your own healthy future.

My dear reader, this is your time to work the book. You have what it takes, so please continue the journey I've laid out for you. Find like-minded people, a coach, or a mentor, and get ongoing support, because one book is not enough. Go to turningfatintolove.com for more free resources after you have finished reading this book.

Thank you for your courage to step out of your old self, for your commitment to change, and for unzipping your old costume and making the decision to step out of it and help others as well by becoming a role model.

With your change you can inspire people around you to do the same, so spread the love, spread the health. Let us turn fat into love and transform lives.

Just like the power of the sun drives the seasons, transforming the world, the power of our heart, and our whole mind drives us through all the seasons of life, transforming our body while we age. No matter what season of life we are in, sometimes we forget to connect to that enormous loving and energetic power inside of us. We seek outside ourselves, we are logged out and disconnected, we've forgotten our username or password, and we remain bewildered. No matter what your relationships with other people or with yourself look like now, when you let more love and energy in again just by generating it yourself, you will transform.

I am not saying it is easy. But I am saying it is worth it. It is worth the struggle and the feelings of discomfort. You will be challenged a lot on your journey toward your happiest and healthiest self. But facing your challenges and busting through them will not only inspire others to overcome theirs, but make you feel incredibly good about yourself.

No matter how intensely we are challenged by life, no matter how brokenhearted we are by love, no matter how much pain our body has inflicted on us, we will never lose our power to get up again. Our power to love again, to live fully again, and to learn again is still inside, no matter how terrible the circumstances. We shake our feathers, we do our little dance with fear, and, yes, here we are again, back in the ring, back on the battlefield, back in life. Yes, we stand there now with a stronger heart; yes, with more wisdom in our head; and, yes, with more vitality in our body. Life and love and health tested us, just to see how badly we wanted to get up again, just to watch our response to the challenges. And when we dare to meet these challenges with our eyes open, life and love and health will reward us with more love, more life, and more health. But when we answer their call with nothing but fear, chances are high that the same challenges will come up again and again, until we decide to finally learn the lesson. Failure is the refusal to learn the lessons from past mistakes, while a mistake is just an opportunity for growth and learning. Failing to try will kill success before it is created.

I honestly believe that we gain much wisdom from all our experiences, all our setbacks, and all our problems. When you are in the midst of stressful times you often don't see the pearls emerging, but you keep on watching the puzzles and can't get the pieces together. That is no problem as long as you have faith that a setback is not the end. It is not the end. It is just a painful new beginning, and you will rise. You will rise in love again. You will rise in health again. You will rise in your life again, more lovable, healthier, and more fully alive.

And now, beyond distance, time, reason, place, and logic, we are connected at this moment. We are connected through these words, these words that were written long before you read them, and yet they are meant for you at this moment in your life. At this moment in your life these words are speaking to you, and these words are messengers. These messengers have come to tell you that you are capable of doing anything that you want and that it is your time.

Your future is whispering to you, softly from inside, inviting you to live healthier, begging you to love yourself a lot more, and craving for you to follow and nourish your dreams.

> *Once you realize that the road is the goal*
> *and that you are always on the road,*
> *not to reach a goal, but to enjoy its beauty and wisdom,*
> *life ceases to be a task and becomes natural*
> *and simple, in itself an ecstasy.*
> —Sri Nisargadatta Maharaj

Reaching the goal, the dream, or the destination is not what will bring us happiness.

It is the road. It is the journey. It is rejoicing in victory after a setback. Enjoy every moment and be present. Embark on your journey to your highest self.

I hope you have safe travels, and that you will fly toward your dreams without any of the extra ballast that was holding you back in the past. Writing this book has freed and healed me, and I have reconnected with an abundance of love inside me. I hope you have felt that energy through the pages.

Now go, go, go—free yourself, heal your body, and turn fat into love, because you are so needed. You are loved and encouraged.

Thank you so much for being you.

—Pauline

# ACKNOWLEDGMENTS

Those who have supported, loved, inspired, and mentored me during the writing of this book will always have a big place in my heart. Always. If there was a hole in my heart that food could not fix, you all have healed and filled that hole. I do love you all to the moon and back with my supersized heart, and you will feel that, even without me saying the words.

First of all, I want to thank my parents for their ongoing incredible support while I was going through the hard times of the divorce while writing a book in a foreign language.

Mum, you are the best granny of the world, and I love you. I adore your commitment to give the little ones what they need the most: love and attention. You have been an anchor for them, and your dedication has given me so much freedom as a single mother. I had complete faith that the kids were safe and loved while I could progress in my work.

Daddy, this book begins with you! I have lived my life with your faith, optimism, and love as a never-ending positive source. Without a doubt I have the confidence to follow my dreams because of you. I see your DNA in my kids and I am happy for them; their life will be easier because of it. I love you so much.

Many thanks to my dear sister Martine for her ongoing support and love for my kids.

Tine, Laura, and Sara: the book would not have been possible without your support and belief.

Tine, thank you for making my life more beautiful. You are a beauty inside out, like little Daan said to you: Mooi! We will create lots of beautiful moments in the future together.

Sara, thank you for your friendship. You refueled me so often with your laughter and compassionate ears. You are funny and intelligent and I love you.

Laura, thank you for your ongoing belief in me, even when I stopped believing. I believe in you and I love you.

Lientje, Gunnhild, and Karin, your practical support, friendship, and warmth were incredibly valuable to me. I am very grateful to have you as friends and family.

Thanks to Brendon Burchard for helping me believe in the power of my own voice and for teaching me how to share my message with the world. This expert journey started at Experts Academy!

To Jennifer and Linda, who were the very first women living in the USA to read and like my book, thank you.

Thanks to Amanda Rooker, who has done an incredible job editing this book and correcting my typos or wrong Dutch-to-English translations without losing my authentic voice. I am so grateful for your work!

Thanks to Morgan James Publishing for making my dream a reality. David and Rick, if I had not gone to Author 101 in Las Vegas, an amazing event, nobody in the world could have ever turned fat into love. Thank you so much for your ongoing support and help.

And last but not least: Thanks to my readers who not only inspired me to share my voice with the world, but also to become a better person.

—Pauline

# ABOUT THE AUTHOR

Pauline Kerkhoff is a dietician, nutritionist, and personal development expert who transforms overweight working women, whether single or in a relationship, into the powerful, energetic, and beautiful women they really are. She does this by helping them connect to the enormous power of their own mind and heart so that they feel fullfilled and happy, and by helping them generate more energy in their bodies.

Kerkhoff received her master's degree in health and nutrition from Wageningen University, one of the top universities in the Netherlands. Her scientific background combined with her practical insights from working with her clients and her own life experiences (such as dealing with disease and divorce) have made her an inspirational transformational expert.

For more than fifteen years she has helped hundreds of overweight and obese people lead happier and healthier lives, including those who have had gastric bandings and gastric bypasses. Knowing that real change always happens from the inside out, she believes that self-love and self-leadership are the best tools for transformation, and she does not believe in diets, shakes, pills, or powders. She loves to travel, to connect with people, to write, and to speak.

A devoted single mother, Kerkhoff lives in the Netherlands with her two children, Kiki (born 2007) and Daan (born 2010).

To learn more, visit

**paulinekerkhoff.com or turningfatintolove.com.**

# RESOURCES

I have been inspired and instructed by many people, whose transformative ideas have served as the foundation of this book. This book has been born from a burning desire to inspire you and to serve you, and you might recognize the voices of my mentors behind my words. I am very grateful for their insights, and I think they will help you too to get the best out of yourself.

Never ever stop learning; it will make your life so much better.

Here they are:

Dr. Daniel Amen: www.drdanielamen.com
Barbara de Angelis: www.barbaradeangelis.com
Brendon Burchard: www.brendonburchard.com
Jack Canfield: www.jackcanfield.com
Louise Hay: www.louisehay.com
Lisa Nichols: www.motivatingthemasses.com
Tony Robbins: www.tonyrobbins.com or
    www.robbinsmadanestraining.com
Robin Sharma: www.robinsharma.com
Brian Tracy: www.briantracy.com
Marianne Williamson: www.mariannewilliamson.com

CPSIA information can be obtained at www.ICGtesting.com
Printed in the USA
LVOW02*1449050614

388778LV00002B/3/P